D0324256

COPING WITH HEARING LOSS

COPING WITH HEARING LOSS

A Guide for Adults and Their Families

by Susan V. Rezen, Ph.D. and Carl Hausman

Foreword by Keenan Wynn

National Chairman, Better Hearing Institute

DEMBNER BOOKS · NEW YORK

Dembner Books
Published by Red Dembner Enterprises Corp., 80 Eighth Avenue, New York, N.Y. 10011
Distributed by W. W. Norton & Company, Inc., 500 Fifth Avenue, New York, N.Y. 10110

Library of Congress Cataloging in Publication Data

Rezen, Susan V.
    Coping with hearing loss.

    Includes index.
    1. Deafness.   2. Adjustment (Psychology)
I. Hausman, Carl, 1953-   .   II. Title.
[DNLM: 1. Audiology—popular works.   WV 270 R467c]
RF291.R48   1985   362.4'2   84-23889
ISBN 0-934878-48-X

To

Mr. and Mrs. Victor Rezen

and

Mr. and Mrs. Carl Hausman, Sr.

Foreword

From the age of fifteen till my early forties, my life was loud with the sound of race cars, ORV's (off-road vehicles, usually motorcycles), and hydroplanes. I loved that sound, but it was murder to my ears. Unfortunately I didn't wear hearing protection and the noise undoubtedly contributed to my hearing loss.

Fortunately I got help. For me it was hearing aids. In fact, most of the millions with hearing loss can now benefit medically, surgically, with hearing aids, or through rehabilitation. The tragedy is that many are not aware of this help, or how to take advantage of it. This is why I have committed myself to many public education projects promoting hearing conservation and available hearing help. This book is especially helpful in this regard.

Coping with Hearing Loss is a sensitive treatment of the physical and psychological effects of hearing loss, and how people can cope with them and overcome hearing problems. It is useful for not only those who suspect a hearing problem, but furthers understanding for the families and friends of hard-of-hearing people.

The authors have done an outstanding job in mitigating the stigma of hearing loss and realistically describing what can be done about it. I heartily recommend this book and believe it will inspire many people to seek and obtain help for uncorrected hearing disorders.

Keenan Wynn
National Chairman
Better Hearing Institute

Contents

Illustrations

Introduction

Having a hearing loss means more than just not being able to hear well. It can bring on a wide range of problems that, at first, you might not suspect have any link to your hearing: isolation from family and friends, a feeling of inadequacy in social situations, and a decline in your overall self-image.

Unfortunately, the social and psychological problems that accompany a hearing impairment are not always immediately obvious, and to make matters worse, the people who should be helping you, often do not. Physicians and audiologists (nonmedical hearing specialists) sometimes lack the training and inclination to tackle these particular problems, and therefore may brush aside the vocational, social, and emotional aspects. Dealing with the physical problem, you see, is frequently a rather cut and dried affair, but helping a patient cope with hearing loss is not.

The purpose of this book is to help you and your family cope with that hearing loss. It will touch on matters as practical as communicating with a mumbling bank teller, choosing a hearing aid, and dealing with doctors. It will also explore some more abstract but equally important concepts: how impaired hearing affects the relationship between husband and wife, why people are reluctant to admit that they don't have perfect hearing, and why they are sometimes just as reluctant to do something about it.

Another section will deal with learning how to adjust to, and use, a hearing aid. As you may already have found out, a hearing aid simply can not restore normal hearing, and it takes a certain amount of skill to use one well.

Rehabilitative hearing therapy will also be discussed: what it involves, where it's offered, and how it can turn things around for an unhappy person struggling with the self-imposed isolation of a hearing disability.

One chapter will explain how the ear functions when it is working correctly, and what happens when it is not. In case this seems as though it will be a bit tedious, remember that a problem rarely seems as frightening or puzzling once you understand what is happening. A basic knowledge of the ear is also helpful when dealing with doctors, audiologists, and hearing aid dispensers.

Medical terms are explained as you read along. In addition, the Glossary at the end of the book will tell you the meaning and pronounciation of these and other terms that may be unfamiliar to you.

It is most important to remember that you are not alone. Hearing loss affects about sixteen million Americans; about half of those people are under the age of sixty-five.

Throughout, this book will trim away the fat and serve up only the lean—the practical knowledge gathered by helping thousands of people learn to live and listen in spite of their hearing loss. There is only one requirement on your part: You have to want to help yourself. To adjust to a hearing aid you must practice an entirely new way of listening, and to cope with reduced hearing you must be willing to change some of your attitudes and behavior. All this can only be accomplished after you admit to yourself that there is a problem and decide to confront it.

But since you picked up this book in the first place—and are still reading it—you're already well on your way.

[1]
Why Am I Losing
My Hearing?

Ears, unfortunately, are somewhat like automobiles: They can malfunction, can be damaged, and often just wear out.

In some cases, disease or heredity conspire to rob the hearing mechanism of its function. Many of us suffer noise damage to the ears, often from exposure to machinery or firearms. Most adults with a hearing impairment have an age-related hearing loss—meaning that as they grew older, their hearing mechanism lost some of its former ability to pick up and transmit sound.

Age-related hearing loss will happen to almost everyone—it just affects some sooner than others. If we all lived to be a hundred and fifty, everyone would have a hearing loss. For many, loss of hearing begins at age fifty-five, but some people forty-five and younger show the symptoms. Hearing loss due to disease or noise damage can occur at any age, but often compounds the problems encountered due to the aging process.

An age-related hearing loss, known scientifically as *presbycusis*, is not medically dangerous, nor is it a symptom of senility or any mental problem. Because there is no way for you to be sure that your hearing loss stems from presbycusis, it is important to see a physician, who can diagnose your problem with a painless examination. It is essential that you see a doctor immediately if your hearing loss comes on suddenly, or is accompanied by pain, dizziness, severe ringing or roaring sensations, a feeling of pressure, or drainage from the ear. These symptoms could indicate a medically significant condition, such as a metabolic imbalance, a circulatory problem, or other disease.

As part of your examination, a physician will probably have your hearing evaluated by an *audiologist*, a communication specialist who tests hearing, recommends hearing aids, and provides counseling and therapy to help clients deal with a hearing disability. Both the physician (either your family doctor or an ear, nose, and throat specialist) and the audiologist will probably use terms that are unfamiliar to you, which is one more reason to

17

arm yourself in advance with some background into the workings of the marvelous mechanism of the ear.

By understanding the ear's function, you will also have a better grasp of what can go wrong with it, and how this situation can be helped. Also, a thorough understanding of what is happening can ease some of the perfectly natural apprehension you feel when something inside you is not working quite right. Let's take a look at the structure of an ear, as shown in Figure 1.

The ear is divided into three parts: the outer ear, middle ear, and inner ear. The outer ear consists of the pinna (the structure of skin and cartilage that hangs on the side of your head) and the ear canal, which extends about an inch into the head.

The human pinna serves as a collector of sound, although not a particularly efficient one. Many animals, dogs for example, have movable pinnas that point in the direction of the sound; some members of the fox family have pinnas so large and mobile that they can detect the sound of ants moving underground.

From the pinna, the sound enters the ear canal, which serves two basic purposes. It protects the fragile eardrum from the elements, and also increases the loudness of certain pitches that are important for understanding speech. These particular pitches are enhanced in the canal by resonance, much the same way in which the sound of your breath is amplified when you blow over the top of a soda bottle.

The middle ear is made up of the eardrum, ossicles, and the eustachian tube. The eardrum (called a tympanum in medical terminology) is a delicate, pearly-white membrane stretched tightly over the end of the ear canal. The eardrum is highly sensitive to vibration, and sound is nothing more than a vibration in the air. After the eardrum picks up this vibration, it passes it along to the ossicles, three tiny bones called the hammer (malleus), anvil (incus), and stirrup (stapes). The ossicles amplify the intensity of the vibration by taking the movement of the comparatively large eardrum and compressing it, so that all the vibration is focused on the minuscule footplate of the stirrup.

This ingenious internal amplifier works best in an air-filled environment, which is provided by the eustachian tube. This tube opens on one end in the middle ear, and on the other end in the back of the throat. It allows

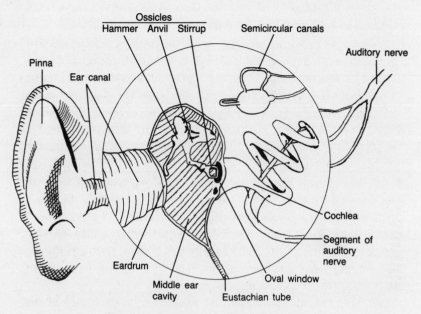

Figure 1: The structure of the human ear

replacement of air absorbed by tissues in the middle ear, drains off fluids that accumulate inside, and provides a way to equalize air pressures inside and outside of the middle ear. The sensation of the tube opening is often felt when your ears "pop" as you ride up an elevator or climb a steep hill.

The inner ear consists of the cochlea (the Latin word for snail), the semicircular canals, and the endings of the auditory nerve. The base of the cochlea and the footplate of the stirrup meet at what's called the oval window, a tissue-covered opening that separates the middle and inner ear and transmits vibration. There is another tissue-covered opening called the round window, which equalizes pressure by moving out when the oval window is pressed in to the inner ear by the footplate of the stirrup.

The intense vibration of the footplate sets up a wave in the fluid filling the cochlea. This wave sets in motion tiny hairlike projections inside the cochlea, which are in contact with the nerve endings. These hair cells, as they are called, translate this motion into nerve impulses, which are carried though the acoustic nerve. This nerve brings the signals to the brain for processing. The semicircular canals do not affect hearing, but they do help you maintain balance by sensing the position of the fluid inside them, giving your body a method to tell if it is level, even if your eyes are closed.

A number of problems can arise within the entire hearing mechanism. One of the most common difficulties is the accumulation of wax (called *cerumen*) in the ear canal. If the ear is plugged with wax, sound cannot travel through it as well. This condition often is brought about when people try to clean their ears. So don't try and clean out the ear canal; just wash the outside of the ear with a washcloth. Any efforts to clean the inside of the ear usually will only make matters worse by pushing the wax farther into the ear canal and impacting it. The ear normally has a mechanism to clean itself, although this mechanism can and does malfunction. Check with your doctor if you think there is too much wax in your ears; a physician is able to remove wax quickly, safely, and painlessly.

Another relatively common problem is a perforated eardrum, that is, a hole in the eardrum, as a result of injury or infection. Such a perforation will probably allow a mucous fluid to drain out of the ear canal, and will allow germs to enter, causing frequent infections.

The space behind the eardrum, the middle ear, is the source of most childhood earaches and infections, but adults can have such problems as well. You know the "plugged" feeling you get in your ears during a cold? Well, the problem is the swelling in your throat, a swelling that restricts the opening of the eustachian tube. When air can't get up the eustachian tube, a slight vacuum is formed in the middle ear. This draws the fluid from the tissues into the middle ear. The fluid alone is enough to cause a problem, but if that fluid gets infected you're in for a bout of *otitis media* (middle ear infection or inflammation) that can be annoying and even painful.

There are several other problems that can crop up in the middle ear. One of the three bones, the stirrup, can have a bony growth around it. This growth "cements" the stirrup in place so that the vibrations are not properly passed to the inner ear. This happens mostly in women and is made worse by pregnancy.

All of these problems cause what's called a *conductive hearing loss*, meaning that the outer or middle ear does not conduct sound as well as it should. The result of a conductive loss is primarily a loss of sensitivity for hearing soft sounds; once sound is loud enough, though, it can be heard adequately.

Now, let's move farther into the head. The inner ear is a very fragile organ, and there are several things that can go wrong with it. One of the inner ear's worst enemies is excessive exposure to noise. Noise exposure causes the tiny hair cells to be banged around, and the violent waves produced by huge vibrations will eventually cause the hair cells to break.

Because a proper supply of oxygen is crucial for the health of the inner ear, problems with circulation (high blood pressure, arteriosclerosis, thrombosis, coronary conditions) can contribute to a hearing loss. Metabolic imbalances such as thyroid problems and diabetes can affect hearing. A common problem is Meniere's disease (also called *endolymphatic hydrops*), where there is too much inner-ear fluid. Meniere's disease can cause a fluctuating hearing loss, a feeling of fullness in the ears, severe dizzy spells, and ringing in the ears.

Speaking of diseases, the inner ear is subject to infection by a variety of viruses, which are often blamed for sudden losses where no other cause is evident. These types of viruses are specific to the inner ear, but other ailments affecting the entire body can also cause a hearing loss. Mumps and measles, for instance, are sometimes responsible; actually, any disease accompanied by an extremely high fever can damage the hearing mechanism.

Further along the tract leading from the ear up to the brain, there is the possiblity of tumors, but this is a very rare condition and is accompanied by other medical symptoms besides hearing loss.

How does age affect the hearing mechanism? For one thing, many components of the ear stiffen up over the years. The joints between the ossicles, for example, stiffen just as knees and elbows do. In the cochlea, there may be stiffening as well as some deterioration of the hair cells; nerve pathways may also degenerate somewhat, and the signal from the ear might not be transmitted clearly to the brain.

When changes from disease, injury, or age occur in the inner ear, they sometimes bring about what's called "nerve deafness." Unfortunately, this term is quite misleading. Nerve deafness not only has nothing to do with being nervous, but the person is also not completely deaf; the loss may be of any degree of severity. What we call nerve deafness refers to damage or destruction of mechanisms in the cochlea and auditory nerve, causing reduced sensitivity to sounds and difficulty in understanding speech. Doctors call this a *sensorineural hearing loss*.

This type of hearing problem, whether we term it nerve deafness or sensorineural hearing loss, can cause decreased capacity in either one or both of two distinct abilities: *sensitivity* to sounds and *discrimination*.

Sensitivity involves the ability to detect soft sounds. People with a sensitivity loss may not be able to hear a whisper or a bird singing, but once the sound is loud enough for them they can interpret it correctly. *Discrimination* refers to the ability to clearly distinguish one sound from another; discrimination is the ability that allows understanding of speech. People with a discrimination problem as well as a sensitivity problem will find that even if speech is made loud enough for them to hear, they will still misunderstand what is being said. Most sensorineural hearing losses involve various combinations of sensitivity and discrimination problems.

Sensitivity is measured in decibels, a rather complicated measurement of loudness. Instead of trying to explain the mathematical definition of a decibel, let's look at the decibel measurements of some common sounds to get an idea of what we are talking about.

0 decibels	The softest sound a typical ear can hear
20 decibels	A whisper
45 decibels	Soft conversational speech
55 decibels	Loud conversational speech
65 decibels	Loud music from a radio
75 decibels	City traffic
100 decibels	A loud factory
110 decibels	A loud amplified rock band
120 decibels	A chain saw or other loud power tool
140 decibels	A jet engine at takeoff

Now that we're on speaking terms with decibel levels, let's turn this example around and observe how a *loss* of a certain amount of hearing affects communication. For example, a person with a 50-decibel loss obviously can not hear sounds that have a loudness of 50 decibels or less, and will therefore have trouble with even loud conversational speech.

A loss of hearing from 1 to 15 decibels is not considered a problem. Proceeding from that point:

Decibel Loss	Hearing Problem
16–25	A slight loss only causes problems if the listening conditions are very poor, as at a noisy party.
26–40	A loss of from 26 to 40 decibels is considered a mild hearing loss. Good communication is possible in ideal listening situations, but background noise and distant speech will be hard to hear. Part-time use of a hearing aid (hearing aids will be discussed in Chapter 6) will be helpful.
41–55	Moderate hearing loss. Conversation can be heard at a distance of three to five feet, but understanding speech is usually a strain, especially in background noise. Full-time use of a hearing aid is necessary.
56–70	Moderately severe hearing loss. Conversation must be very loud and nearby to be understood, and very little can be heard in group situations. A hearing aid is needed, but may not be the whole solution at times. Speechreading instruction (to be dealt with in Chapter 11) and speech therapy and counseling (to be dealt with in Chapter 12) are helpful.
71–90	Severe hearing loss. Only very loud speech, about one foot away from the ear, can be heard, and it is often quite distorted. A hearing aid will provide some benefit, but speechreading training and counseling are also needed. Work with a speech therapist may be needed to keep speech from deteriorating (speech sounds may become distorted when the speaker can not hear himself correctly).
91 or more	Profound hearing loss, or deafness. Some very loud sounds may be heard (or felt through vibration). Training in speechreading, speech therapy, and counseling are absolutely essential.

One dilemma caused by sensitivity losses, even mild ones, is that they frequently are most severe at higher pitches, or more correctly, higher frequencies. Many consonants are high-pitched sounds formed by air exploding or hissing from the mouth, such as *f, s, v, sh, th, ch, p, k, z,* and *t*. When the ear can't properly receive these high-frequency sounds, words like "Sue," "chew," and "shoe" may all sound the same, and the context of the sentence must be used to fill in the missing sounds. Even if you can't hear the *sh* in "I've got a hole in my shoe," you can still figure out what was said by the meaning of the rest of the sentence. However, if you must figure out too many words from context, the task becomes too difficult and the conversation can not be followed. Soon, it becomes difficult to determine if you really can't hear or whether you are just "tuning out."

Now let's consider discrimination, and how it affects communication. This ability to distinguish one sound from another is measured by determining what percentage of a list of one-syllable words can be correctly recognized when presented at a comfortable loudness (this test will be explained in greater detail in Chapter 8). Identifying individual words is harder than picking them up in a conversation, however, so keep in mind that a discrimination score of 90 percent means that you can pick out more than nine out of ten words during a conversation.

Ninety-percent discrimination, by the way, is considered the lower limit for normal hearing, meaning that someone at this level will have hardly any problem communicating, assuming that speech is presented loudly enough to eliminate any trouble caused by a loss of sensitivity. When the discrimination ability drops below normal, these problems arise:

Discrimination Ability	Hearing Problem
75–90%	Mild difficulty understanding speech, especially in background noise. The mind is able, though, to fill in the gaps and figure out what was said in most situations.
60–75%	Moderate difficulty in communication. Speech often seems distorted, and it is difficult to follow a conversation.
45–60%	Moderately severe difficulty communicating. Techniques such as speechreading must be used to fill in the gaps and understand what is being said.
Below 45%	Speech sounds like a foreign language, and there is severe difficulty in communication.

Just amplifying the loudness of the sound does not necessarily help a discrimination problem, although when there is also a drop in sensitivity, a hearing aid can be beneficial.

There is no way for you to accurately test your own hearing, but it's safe to assume that if you think you have a loss, you probably do, and should have your hearing evaluated. If you're not sure about whether you have a hearing problem (remember, it can sneak up over a period of years and is not always obvious to you), try asking yourself a few questions.

- Do I tune out from conversations where there is more than one person talking?
- Am I letting my spouse or my best friend do most of my talking for me?
- After a long conversation, am I usually tired and irritable?
- When I answer people's questions, do they often appear puzzled or embarrassed by my response?
- Does it seem that my friends and family are avoiding conversation with me?
- Do I frequently misunderstand people, and ask them to repeat what they have said?

If you answered yes to one or more of these questions, it's possible that you have a hearing loss, one that you may not even be conscious of. An evaluation by an audiologist can determine whether your particular hearing loss is worse at certain frequencies, whether it involves sensitivity or discrimination loss (or both), and how bad your loss is.

Although this short course in the nature of a hearing loss leaves a lot of ground uncovered, it should have provided you with enough background to understand your hearing loss and discuss it with a doctor or audiologist. There are certainly some questions you would still like answered, so we'll deal with a few of the most commonly asked questions that come up at this point.

How much worse will my hearing loss become? Unfortunately, there is no way to make an accurate prediction. Recent research has shown that some age-related hearing losses stabilize around the age of sixty-five, though there's no guarantee of that happening. If your loss is due to noise exposure, you can prevent further damage by staying out of the noise, or by using earmuffs or earplugs to reduce the intensity of the noise. Progression of losses due to heredity or disease will vary with the specific cause. The best tactic is to have your hearing tested every two years after your initial visit to a doctor and audiologist. If there is a change, your hearing should be tested more frequently after that.

Why me, and not my friends who are the same age? Some of them hear very well. Some people are predisposed toward a hearing loss, just as some people are more likely to gain weight, have heart trouble, or develop high blood pressure. Heredity plays a part, so if your parents developed presbycusis at an early age, you may have inherited a tendency toward it. Exposure to noise, such as years of work in a foundry, can also hasten the effects of an oncoming loss. Your general health, now and through your entire life, also plays a role in determining how well your hearing will hold up in later years.

Is it permanent? Yes, except for a few cases that will respond to medical or surgical treatment (explained in Chapter 7).

I sometimes have a ringing in my ears. Am I going crazy? Hardly. Tinnitus, a ringing, roaring, or clicking sensation in the ears, affects millions. These sounds often accompany hearing loss, although their source is usually unknown, and medical science has not found a cure. However, there are methods to help alleviate tinnitus (discussed in Chapter 10).

Not only can tinnitus obscure speech sounds, making understanding difficult, it can also cause so much distraction and distress that concentrating on what is being said is almost impossible.

You talk about going to see a doctor or an audiologist. Which one should I see first? It really doesn't matter, since you will almost certainly have to see both. A doctor will refer you to an audiologist, and if the doctor you see is an ear, nose, and throat specialist, an audiologist may be there on the staff. An audiologist will want you to see a doctor to make sure there is no medical problem. In most cases, it will probably be simplest to see the doctor first.

Can drugs I am taking affect my hearing? Yes, in some cases. Aspirin or drugs with aspirin in them, taken in high doses (usually ten pills a day or more), can temporarily diminish hearing. Quinine, which is sometimes prescribed for muscle cramps, can also have a temporary effect. Such losses are usually preceded by tinnitus, so if such symptoms arise you should consult the doctor who prescribed the medication. Certain powerful antibiotics, used only to combat a life-threatening infection, can cause a permanent hearing loss, but the law requires that you be told if one of these *ototoxic* (dangerous to hearing) drugs are prescribed.

Now that you have a better understanding of the nature of hearing loss, you will be better prepared to cope with it, and move onto the next chapter—an examination of the way a hearing loss can shape the way you feel about yourself and the people around you.

[2]
The Psychological Effects
of a Hearing Loss

Millions of people go through needless emotional suffering simply because they have not been adequately prepared to cope with their hearing disability. Professionals in the hearing field, who may be experts at treating the physical side of a hearing loss, often don't have the time or motivation to explain and help deal with a client's typical anxieties and emotions.

In the case of an age-related hearing disability, for example, the psychological effects that go hand in hand with the physical problem are just as much a natural part of the aging process as the hearing loss itself. When these emotional reactions are not dealt with properly they can be magnified all out of proportion, and may even cause drastic personality and lifestyle changes.

Psychologists have found that almost everyone who endures an emotional or physical loss goes through the same stages of *denial, projection, anger, depression,* and *acceptance.* Let's examine the impact of these emotional stages on someone who is trying to adjust to a hearing loss.

Denial is a natural initial reaction if you are faced with a threat to your physical or emotional well-being, because it is painful to accept at first, and your emotions seek a way to stall for time to muster the resources to accept this unpleasant fact. At first, it's easy to deny a hearing loss, because it may build up so gradually that it is not perceptible. The denial stage, though, can be—and often is—carried to extremes. A wife, for example, may point out to her husband that during the party they just left he didn't catch most of the conversation. "Nonsense," he replies. "I just didn't want to listen to that old windbag." An attitude like this will eventually lead to friction between husband and wife, or among family members. Eventually, though, even the most stubborn person must realize that there is a problem, one that will not go away because it is ignored. Still, the mind may not be ready to accept a permanent hearing loss, and will still confront the situation bit by bit.

Projection is the next emotional safety valve after denial, and involves blaming your problem on someone else. "Speak up! Why the hell do you

31

mumble all the time?" Remember, though, that there may frequently be some other basis for projection, in addition to your need for a defense mechanism. A commonly heard type of projection is the complaint that "young people nowadays mumble terribly." Well, to a certain extent this is true; without question, there is less attention paid to elocution by our modern school system. However, a person with normal hearing would not have as much trouble understanding a mumbling teenager as would someone with a hearing loss, so it is not logical to conclude that your *entire* problem in understanding people stems from the way they talk.

Anger usually follows projection, and may take two forms: a generalized "mad at the world" resentment, and a specific anger directed toward an individual, usually the one with whom the hearing-impaired person spends the most time. An attitude of continual anger will strain even the strongest relationship, but once again we have to bear in mind that anger in this case may have some basis in reality. A spouse or family member must be careful not to go overboard in pointing out the social blunders of a hearing-impaired person, because that type of continual criticism will just bring about more anger. (Chapter 5 will specifically address this problem.)

Depression comes after all anger is vented, and can often be accompanied by acute embarrassment over past behavior, along with isolation and a personality change; an abrupt personality change may leave friends and family rather frightened of this "new person" in their midst, thus heightening the feeling of isolation felt by the hearing-impaired person.

Again, remember that there is a *very real* reason for this depression, and one aspect of the cause usually is not even considered by family and friends: There is often a "dead feeling" that comes from not hearing background noise, the sounds that those with perfect hearing take for granted. Someone with even a mild hearing loss may be saddened— consciously or unconsciously—by the fact that birds no longer chirp, downtown no longer hums, and the wind has stopped whistling through the trees.

We also rely on hearing to warn us of impending threats, such as someone approaching from behind, or tampering with the back door. It is quite natural for these feelings of insecurity to aggravate a general depression, and encourage withdrawal and suspicion.

Although this typical depression is understandable, it is far from desirable, and while it probably will happen, at least briefly, to everyone who experiences hearing loss, in some people this emotional stage can linger for years, becoming a virtual life sentence of isolation. Only after chronic depression is seen for what it is—self-imposed exile from the human race—can it be conquered.

Acceptance comes after the depression has lifted, and involves the realization that "there is something wrong with my hearing, not with *me.*" This is the only stage where the problems of hearing loss can really be dealt with effectively.

How long does it take to get to the acceptance stage? It's hard to say. For some it may be a matter of days or weeks, while others may need years. But for most it seems to be a matter of months before the realization of a hearing loss can be digested, so the speak. It is important to bear in mind that until you have completely accepted your hearing loss, getting a hearing aid may be futile, or even counterproductive.

You probably have noticed that up until this point hearing aids have been mentioned only in passing, and won't be completely covered until Chapter 6. The reason for this is to avoid giving you the impression that a hearing aid is the only factor in coping with a hearing loss.

Although it is very important, a hearing aid is not a cure-all, nor will it restore all of your lost hearing. Using the aid properly will require diligent practice for the first few weeks of its use. It is essential that a hearing aid user be emotionally ready to cope with the hearing loss and with the difficulties of using the aid. Simply getting a hearing aid will *not* solve your problems.

Many of you wear hearing aids at this point, and are reading this book because you want information on how to use the aid properly. If you have adjusted to your hearing impairment and accepted the fact that you must work to cope with it, the material on better listening habits will benefit you greatly.

Some of you have worn hearing aids in the past, but have since stuck them in the dresser drawer because you were sorely disappointed in their performance (and you probably never received proper instruction and counseling in their use, either). An examination of your emotions at the time you stopped using your aid will probably be very helpful to you.

Most of the readers of this book picked it up in the first place because of an interest in getting a first hearing aid, or another, better-suited one. If you fall into this category, you would be wise to take inventory of your feelings and be sure that you are completely prepared to admit that you need a hearing aid and are prepared to learn how to use it. Otherwise, an initial bad experience may rob you of motivation that might never be recaptured.

What might be holding you back? It's possible that you still attach a stigma to wearing a hearing aid. Even though people will wear eyeglasses to correct a slight deviation in their vision, they often will resist wearing a hearing aid, although they may need it badly.

Perhaps this relates to the fact that many young people wear glasses, and therefore glasses are not viewed as a sign of an age-related disability. Neither should hearing aids—and as you will see in later chapters, most hearing aids are practically invisible, anyway.

Maybe you are not yet emotionally ready. It takes time to adjust, certainly, but some people linger in the same stage (usually depression) for years. This usually happens because they did not comprehend what was happening to them emotionally when they were passing through the typical stages following a hearing loss, and therefore *could not cope with feelings that they did not understand.*

It all boils down to learning from the experience of others. Millions of people have been through the same situation you are now facing, and most make it through successfully—but not without their share of mistakes, self-doubt, and anxiety. Imagine how much easier it would have been, had they been prepared for those emotional difficulties they would encounter along the way! They could have been spared many of the deep-seated suspicions that typically come along in such cases—suspicions that they were becoming senile, or seriously ill, or emotionally disturbed.

Our next topic will be an examination of just how these emotional stages affect relationships among family members. First, there are some commonly asked questions concerning the psychological effects of hearing loss that you still may wish answered.

Those emotional stages are interesting, but how can I tell which one I'm in? It's not all that simple, because these phases are general guidelines and not specific milestones in your psychological process. However, you can get a reasonable idea of where you stand by observing what you do and say when your hearing impairment causes a problem. Here are some typical actions and statements that indicate various stages:

Denial

- Pretending that you heard what was said, giving an inappropriate answer, and then ignoring the fact that your answer didn't make sense to the person with whom you are speaking.
- Claiming a lack of interest or attention when that's really not the case. "I can hear when I want to listen."

Projection

- "The acoustics of this room are lousy."
- "Why can't my nephew learn to stop mumbling?"

Anger

- "If you're ashamed to be seen with me, why don't you go by yourself?"
- "I hate those Smiths! We had a terrible time at dinner last night, and I won't go out with them again."

Depression

- "I've been making a fool out of myself in front of the Smiths because of this stupid hearing problem, and I'll never be able to face them again."
- "Everything seems so dead, I might as well be dead, too."

Acceptance

- "I don't want to miss out on things any more."
- "Even if I can't hear very well, I can still see and think, and my health is still good."

How do I know if I have been in a particular stage too long? It has been too long if the characteristics of a particular stage are harming your lifestyle, personality, or relationships with other people. In other words, you know you're not making much progress when your emotions control *you*, instead of the other way around.

What should I do if I am not making progress? Seek professional help, ideally an audiologist with experience in dealing with the social and psychological effects of hearing loss. If you feel capable of it, you can try and work out your own problems, which may be easier now that you have some insight into the nature of a hearing loss and the range of its effects.

I feel that I have pretty well accepted my problem, and want to get it taken care of eventually. Is there any rush? Yes. Quite often, people reach the acceptance stage but don't take action, and as a result may slip back into other, less productive attitudes. If you feel ready, you should do it now, and the step-by-step course of action you should take will be outlined later in this book.

My hearing loss seemed to become a major problem right after I retired. Why? Retirement can be very traumatic. In effect, it's like being told you suddenly can't do the things you were capable of before reaching retirement age. A hearing loss can be a constant reminder that you're "not what you used to be." It's no wonder that the hearing loss seems worse when coupled with an unwelcome retirement.

Retirement also means that you will be spending more time with your spouse, family, or close friends, and your hearing loss affects *them*, also. The next chapter will explain why you and your family must be aware of your feelings to insure that actions are not misinterpreted, causing a strain on relationships.

[3]
How a Hearing Loss Can
Ruin a Relationship

We don't always have the power to see ourselves as we really are. Counselors are aware of how difficult it is for some clients to describe a situation in which they are directly involved. To overcome this difficulty, case histories are often presented, because most people find it easier to recognize their own behavior when seen in the actions of others.

It is valuable to recognize certain behaviors, especially the ones you want to change. You can't change something until you know what you're dealing with. These case histories of actual relationships affected by hearing loss may throw some light on the matter. See if you recognize yourself.

Case History 1

Depression and Withdrawal. Sally was tolerant. She withstood the blaming and anger of her husband, Arthur, from the onset of his hearing loss. "He's changed," Sally said, "but he's still my husband, and I have to learn to live with this."

When Arthur reached the depression stage, he felt terribly guilty about his treatment of Sally. He began to hate himself for it, feeling that he didn't deserve such a tolerant woman. "She would be better off without me," Arthur felt—and he eventually withdrew into a shell, removing himself from her life.

Sally was bewildered. She couldn't imagine what she had done to make Arthur dislike her (which is how it appeared to her). As a result, she also became depressed and withdrawn.

Case History 2

The Tower of Strength. Frank, a policeman, had always been a powerful and dominant figure in his family; Bea, his wife, and their two children depended on him heavily. But when Frank began to struggle through the typical problems that come with hearing loss, Bea and the children became terrified, because their tower of strength was beginning to crumble. "He's always been so self-confident and capable," she thought, "but he's changed. Where does this leave us?"

Bea began to spend more time with relatives and friends, looking for comfort—and someone else to depend on. The boys spent more and more time away from home. Frank, meanwhile, felt deserted. Just when he really needed help from his family, they weren't there.

Case History 3

Continual Confrontation. Evelyn had a hearing loss, and she was mad at the world. Because she was angry almost all the time, life at home was not too pleasant, which made husband Joe angry, too.

Joe began to nag. "You didn't hear a word they said at that party. You made me feel like a fool."

Joe's attitude only made Evelyn angrier. The two fought, literally, every moment they spent together. Because of this situation, Evelyn never did anything about her problem. Why? Because she was angry at Joe, and knew in her own odd way that her hearing problem was the best way to "get back at him," by making him miserable, too.

Case History 4

Passive Aggression. Vivian was mad at the world, too—but she is a quiet woman who wouldn't dream of "making a scene" about the hearing loss of her husband, Cliff.

If Cliff has a hearing loss, why is Vivian angry? Even she probably is not sure, but the conditions that soured the relationship almost certainly existed long before Cliff's hearing began to fade. When Cliff's loss became obvious, Vivian used it as a way to vent her subtle anger.

She spoke very softly, even though Cliff was hardly ever able to hear her the first time. In many cases she would speak with her head turned, and Cliff would become extremely frustrated because he just couldn't understand what was being said.

Vivan is not an aggressive complainer, but she found a quiet and diabolically effective way to take out her long-standing anger on Cliff.

Case History 5

Drifting Apart. Agnes and Randall always thought of themselves as the perfect couple, and in many ways they were. The two had survived thirty years of marriage with few quarrels, and it seemed as though they would sail on smooth waters forever.

But when Randall began to experience the emotional problems that accompany hearing loss, he found himself unable to express his feelings to Agnes. "I just can't talk about things like that," he had always felt.

Unlike other couples, they didn't bicker. They didn't blame. They just began to live separate lives under one roof. Randall felt somewhat ashamed of his "weakness," and Agnes began to feel the same way, too. While they never showed any outward signs of conflict, they had stopped communicating—and neither was very happy.

Case History 6

Suffocating with Kindness. Ellie always thought of herself as the strong one in her marriage with Alfred. She had always handled all the problems, so why shouldn't she rise to the challenge of Alfred's hearing loss?"

Unfortunately, Ellie's idea of help was to take over Alfred's life, and the hearing problem (which Ellie didn't like to talk about) just made things worse. When Alfred, in a period of projection, would say, "The people at that meeting mumbled so badly I couldn't catch a word," Ellie would *agree* with him, even though she knew it wasn't true.

She thought she was protecting her husband, and acted with the best of intentions, but she was really suffocating him. Even though Alfred might want to go to a party, she would avoid it. "You know you won't like it, Al, so let's just stay home." Still, she would never admit that her husband's problems stemmed from a hearing loss. In effect, she put Alfred in a position where he could not face up to his hearing problem—he couldn't even admit to having one, because his strong-willed wife denied it.

Alfred stayed quiet, but resentful, unable to come to grips with his hearing loss.

Case History 7

Confronting Mortality. Paul, a widower, really enjoyed visits from his son and grandchildren. Lately, though, those visits had been few and far between.

Paul's hearing loss really didn't bother him that much; but his forty-year-old son, Paul Junior, just couldn't cope with it.

Paul Junior just could not handle the fact that his father was getting older. "Dad just isn't the same. He's not himself. I can't stand to see him this way."

True, Paul Senior had his problems, but—at first—he regarded his hearing loss as a natural part of the aging process, and nothing to be afraid or ashamed of. So why didn't his son feel the same way?

Paul Junior wasn't really reacting to his father's hearing loss. He was upset because his father was getting older and wouldn't be around forever. (And this also brought home the point that Paul Junior was getting older, too.) Father had always been a stable pillar in young Paul's life, and the hearing loss seemed to point up the fact that no one lives forever.

But Father didn't understand all this. He thought his son was snubbing him because of his hearing problem. Paul Senior became increasingly hurt, angry, and depressed.

Case History 8

Patronizing a Parent. Hal, a successful junior executive, decided that his mother, Clara, was getting senile. "She can hardly carry on a conversation," Hal said. "I've got to start taking care of her. After all, she took care of me for years."

Clara, in the beginning, really didn't feel disabled. She did have some trouble communicating, even with her hearing aid, but did her best to cope.

When Hal began to take over her life, though, her self-image began to change. "Well, maybe there is something wrong with me, or Hal wouldn't act like this."

Eventually, Clara let herself be molded into the role of a weak, dependent old woman—even though she hated it and resented Hal for forcing the role on her.

* * *

You probably have noticed that all the people in these case histories experienced problems because they (or someone close to them) were mired in a stage of denial, projection, anger, or depression. If these psychological stages seemed a bit abstract when they were explained in the previous chapter, perhaps they struck home in the case histories—which is exactly why they were presented.

Before moving on, let's review some of the more common questions about the effects of a hearing loss on a relationship.

I don't seem to fit completely into any of those case histories, but I do recognize myself in bits and pieces of several. Is this normal? Of course. Not every situation can be pigeonholed into a particular category, and situations are also affected by the personalities of individuals, as well as the condition of the relationship before the hearing loss. Perhaps some people would find that none of the case histories applied.

If the brief descriptions were illuminating, try writing down a similar paragraph or two describing your particular situation. At the risk of being repetitious, we remind you: You can not change something until you know what it is you want to change.

In the example of Clara and her son, you mentioned that her son thought she was senile. What exactly is senility? It is the physical deterioration of nerve and brain tissue, which is sometimes complicated by inadequate circulation to these tissues. This condition causes problems in memory and abstract thinking. Clara certainly wasn't senile—she just had problems communicating.

Is senility less common than most laymen believe? Yes. Often, problems in communication brought on by hearing loss are mistaken for senility, especially by people who bandy the word about, without really knowing what it means. In some cases, what seems to be senility has been induced by the assortment of drugs sometimes given to older people.

My situation seems so bad that I don't see how it can ever be improved. What can I do? Things may not be as bad as they seem, but to be perfectly honest, relationships sometimes do deteriorate to the point where they are irreconcilable. If, after reading the next chapter, you still don't see a light at the end of the tunnel, it is advisable to seek professional help, such as a psychologist, marriage and family therapist, or an audiologist. (Be sure to determine, as best you can, that your psychologist or therapist is interested in and has some knowledge of hearing loss; conversely, if you visit an audiologist be sure that he or she is concerned with rehabilitative counseling. Where to find professional help, and how to choose a therapist, are outlined in chapters 8 and 12.)

[4]
If You Have a
Hearing Loss

To risk oversimplifying the situation, let's consider two short statements that can often get directly to the root of problems associated with hearing loss.

It is *your* hearing loss, but it has an effect on everyone around you. It changes your behavior, and therefore alters the way people react to you.

That sounds pretty simple, doesn't it? Yet these points are often ignored, much to the sorrow of many hearing-impaired people who can't understand why things have changed.

Even though things change after a hearing loss, your life doesn't necessarily have to change for the worse. You must be willing to accept the facts that you have a permanent hearing loss and that it will *affect* your life and relationships with others—but the loss does not have to *harm* those relationships. If you can learn from the mistakes of others, there's a very good chance that you can avoid stepping in the same emotional quicksand.

The case histories discussed in the previous chapter were presented with this in mind. Unfortunately, there's no way to say "in Case History 1, Arthur could have solved all his problems by . . ." because human relationships are just too complicated for any pat answers.

However, as we've pointed out, once you've identified what is happening to you it is far easier to deal with; you can use your newly acquired knowledge to develop a healthy attitude about hearing loss and how it may affect your relationships with others. It is also important for you to instill this healthy attitude into those close to you, to insure that they don't sabotage your efforts by clinging to their own negative feelings.

Just what constitutes a healthy attitude? There are plenty of theories (none of them necessarily correct in every case), but these suggestions have proven useful to most people confronted with a hearing loss.

- Be aware that your hearing loss affects other people, and be prepared to deal with their reactions.

- Find out as much as you possibly can concerning hearing loss, both in terms of physical and psychological effects. Learn about ways to help yourself communicate more effectively.
- Recognize emotional factors in yourself. Be willing and able to say, "I'm taking out my anger on my wife because she's the only person who will put up with it" or "I accused my wife of mumbling, but it's really my problem, not hers." You must be willing to make an honest effort to cope with these problems.
- Admit your problem to those around you, and be prepared to discuss it with people who are affected. You must also fully accept the fact that you do have a problem, but also realize that something can be done to help you deal with it.
- Most people are willing and able to help you communicate better, and you should be willing to accept their assistance. But never forget that dealing with hearing loss is *your responsibility*. You can not expect other people to solve your problems, nor can you take out your frustrations on them.

The ultimate goal of coping with a hearing loss is, of course, to feel better about yourself; when that happens, you will improve relations with those around you. Consider, too, that the natural reaction of friends and family, who see you taking positive action, will be favorable—and they will express this attitude by wanting to help you improve even more.

Let's discuss how this positive attitude could help the people we met in Chapter 3:

The *depression and withdrawal* symptoms faced by tolerant Sally and her angry husband, Arthur, probably stemmed from an initial lack of communication. Sally never really understood that her husband was angry *about his hearing loss*, and not angry *at her*. When Arthur became depressed and withdrew, Sally had no way of knowing that his reaction wasn't an expression of dislike for her.

If Arthur had been aware that his hearing loss would affect Sally, and made an effort to deal with her reaction, conditions almost certainly would have been better for both of them.

When strong ex-cop Frank was no longer a *tower of strength* to his wife, she didn't display a healthy attitude (which is important even though it was not her hearing loss). Bea made no effort to learn about hearing loss, to understand that it is not a weakness. Frank didn't help matters much, either; he didn't go out of his way to discuss the problem, or admit that he needed support from his wife (because he thought it would be a sign of weakness).

Both could have coped better if they had recognized their own emotions, owning up to the fact that they were frightened of the "weakness" that they associated with Frank's hearing impairment.

Evelyn and Joe, the unfortunate couple locked in *continual confrontation*, had an unhealthy attitude from the word go. Evelyn should have stopped to consider that her constant anger would have an effect on her husband, making him angry, too; by analyzing her feelings and taking responsibility for her hearing problem, she might have avoided her tragic sin of taking out her anger on someone who cared for her.

Vivian, the specialist in *passive aggression*, made life miserable for her hearing-impaired husband. Because of her attitude, any effort by Cliff to help himself would probably be undermined.

How could a healthy attitude have helped? Remember that there's no quick solution in a case such as this (because this relationship might have been in pretty bad shape even before the hearing loss) but bringing the problem out into the open might be a start. By recognizing emotional factors (Vivian's passive aggression, which may be largely subconscious) the couple would take the first step toward improving their lot, and easing the continual tension between them.

Agnes and Randall, the "perfect couple" who are *drifting apart*, need a better understanding of the nature of a hearing loss and how it is changing their lives.

Alfred, whose wife, Ellie, is *suffocating* him *with kindness*, has a problem accepting responsibility for his hearing loss. While the problem is shared by both of them, it's up to Alfred to declare that he is a whole person who does not want to be trapped in the role of a social invalid.

Would a better attitude have helped ease the parent-child conflicts described in Chapter 3? If Paul Junior, the son who is troubled by *confronting mortality* and can't accept the fact that his father is growing old, could understand the nature of a hearing loss he might be able to tolerate it better. If father Paul knew more about the effects of his hearing loss on his son, Paul would realize that his son is not stopping by as often because of misconceptions and misunderstandings about the hearing impairment (that it indicates frailty or mental derangement). Paul would know that his son still likes him; think how much anguish could be saved by this simple understanding.

Clara, the woman *patronized* by her son Hal, is becoming rapidly convinced that she is a disabled old woman. It's important for Clara to take responsibility for herself, and eliminate debilitating self-doubts. She must convince her well-meaning son that the behavior associated with hearing loss does not indicate incompetence or senility.

Don't forget that bringing about an actual change in behavior is a difficult process—much more complicated then the one- or two-sentence descriptions of what could be accomplished with a healthy attitude. Admittedly, the examples discussed are simplified almost to the point of absurdity; they are presented as illustrations, not step-by-step formulas for personal happiness. There are no such formulas—but the case histories should give you some ideas on how to analyze and confront problems related to your hearing loss.

Experience is an excellent teacher; unfortunately, many of us learn the hard way. The people in the case histories found that dealing with the emotional and social consequences of impaired hearing is actually tougher than facing up to the actual communication problems. That's why so much of this book deals with these complex emotions, in hopes that you can benefit from what others have been through.

Notice that many of the most unhappy people you know suffer from deep-seated resentment—of others, of circumstances, or of their own emotional or medical problems. To be frank, the proverbial "chip on the shoulder" is common among people with poor hearing. Blaming others is convenient for them. It is an easy habit to fall into, but it is always a trap. As we've seen, when you take resentment out on others, *they resent you*, and a vicious cycle is formed.

Here are some of the more common questions asked about the topics covered in this chapter:

If I learn to cope with my hearing loss, can I return to a completely normal life? No matter how well you cope, or how well you adapt to a hearing aid, there are going to be some occupations and activities you just won't be able to handle. However, a hearing loss doesn't have to cripple your lifestyle, and while your life may not be exactly as it always was, it need not be any less worthwhile and rewarding.

How long will it take to make things better? There's no simple answer to that, other than to warn against expecting overnight results.

As far as being able to cope with just the physical aspects, you'll remember that if you don't currently have a hearing aid, you can't expect miracles. If you do have a hearing aid, you probably realize by now that it takes effort and practice.

Where emotions are concerned, remember that new behavior has to be practiced until it becomes a habit (taking the place of past behavior, which was also a habit). Think of people you know who have gone on crash diets, only to gain all that weight back. They failed because they didn't make their new behavior (cutting down food intake) a habit. The same theory applies to coping with a hearing loss: You can't just practice a new kind of behavior once or twice and expect it to become part of your lifestyle.

If you can master that new behavior, you're well on your way to establishing a new outlook, which will benefit you and those close to you. Because the people in your life play such a large part in the way you handle a hearing loss, they should read the next chapter, which is specifically written for them.

[5]
If Your Spouse, Parent, or Friend Has a Hearing Loss

This chapter is written for those who have frequent contact with someone who has a hearing loss—perhaps a spouse, parent, relative, or close friend. Those of you with a hearing loss would be well advised to keep reading, too, because you may gain some insight into how people who are seemingly insensitive to your problem simply may not know any better.

Those of you who do not have a hearing loss: Do you know what it would be like? Chances are, you probably don't. Here's why: You can imagine what it's like to be blind by closing your eyes or turning off the lights, but you can't stop your hearing. Even plugging your ears tightly simulates only a mild hearing loss, and there are distortion factors that normal-hearing people can not duplicate.

Persons with normal hearing also may ask why such a big deal is made of emotional problems in relation to hearing loss (and why three of the first four chapters of this book dealt with it exclusively).

The most effective way to explain is by illustration.

Here are some of the problems faced by the hearing impaired:

- *Frustration*, because they don't understand much of what is being said, and have to ask people to repeat themselves.
- *Fear of embarrassment*, because they make some inappropriate responses during conversation, or make no response at all when one is expected.
- *Tension*, because they must constantly be extremely alert, afraid they will miss something important, or that someone will change the topic and they won't catch on quickly.
- *Exhaustion*, because for them, listening is not a passive activity. It requires that they actively attempt to fill in what they miss, and predict what will be said.

Here are some comparable situations that would make a normal-hearing person experience these feelings:

- *Frustration*: You are buying vegetables at a market in an ethnic neighborhood. You are asking questions of the grocer, who has a very thick accent. Most people around you are speaking a foreign language. You are having a great deal of trouble understanding the grocer, and people behind you in line are growing impatient. The grocer (an arrogant sort of fellow) seems amused that you must continually ask him to repeat himself. He gestures to friends nearby, and says something you do not understand. Everybody—except you—laughs at what the grocer says.

- *Fear of embarrassment*: It's difficult to come up with a directly comparable situation, but you may have experienced this emotion at a party with people you do not know; they may have been part of a different social class, or members of a political or fraternal group you are not part of. When people ask you direct questions, you are afraid of inadvertently offending someone, or displaying ignorance of the topic at hand.

- *Tension*: You are driving to an appointment in an unfamiliar city; you are alone in the car and it is snowing. You are driving slowly—much to the displeasure of drivers behind you—because you are afraid you'll miss a street sign. You're expending no more physical energy than you would driving home from work in your home town, but how do your nerves feel in this situation?

- *Exhaustion*: You've taken someone to a restaurant for a business meeting. As you begin dinner, a rock band (which you didn't know was going to be there when you picked out the restaurant) starts to play—at full blast, of course. You must strain to catch every word, and you find yourself staring at your companion's mouth, trying to get some clue as to what is being said. By the end of the evening, you are tired and irritable. Your pleasant dinner meeting was turned into a real chore because communication was so difficult.

Get the picture? What to you is simple communication is a tiring effort for those with a hearing problem, and the kinds of factors illustrated make it a tedious and trying process. That's why some hearing-impaired people tend to forego communication altogether, or can only tolerate some social situations for a brief period of time.

It is doubly frustrating for the hearing impaired when their families and friends don't understand this. In fact, people with hearing losses often feel (with justification) that they are victims of widespread prejudice and misconception. (It's not unheard of for someone with a hearing loss to use the term "bigot" to describe a person who makes no effort to understand the problem.)

Are you treating someone unfairly? Take this brief quiz and find out. Do you:

- Ever talk as if the hearing-impaired person isn't there?
- Avoid sitting down to carry on a conversation?
- Accuse someone with a hearing loss of only listening when he or she wants to?
- Shout if someone doesn't hear the first time?
- Tell someone to turn up the hearing aid?
- Speak to the person as if he or she were a child?
- Take over responsibility for answering the door or the telephone, without being asked to?

If you answered affirmatively to any of these questions, you might be acting very unfairly. Some of the situations need no explanation, and deal with consideration and manners (talking around or ignoring someone in a conversation), while others involve misconceptions that may lead to inappropriate reactions on your part.

For instance, nothing makes a hearing-impaired person's blood boil faster than the familiar accusation that "you only listen when you want to—you use your hearing as an excuse to tune out when you're not interested." This holds just a kernel of truth: As has been pointed out, listening is an *active* (as opposed to a passive) activity for people with a hearing loss. They must make a special effort to understand. Whether they understand often hinges on a complex mixture of listening conditions, background noise, and the voice of the person speaking; if you take the time to sit down and analyze each particular situation, there will be definite reasons why someone can hear in some situations, but not in others. Yes, it sometimes depends on interest—but if you had to make a tiring effort every time you had to listen, wouldn't you "tune out" from time to time?

Equally rankling is the command to "turn up your hearing aid if you can't understand!" First of all, most people with an age-related hearing loss have problems with both sensitivity and discrimination (see Chapter 1) and often hear speech as distorted sound. *Turning up the volume can not make distorted sound any clearer, and may actually make the situation worse.* Overly loud sound coming through the hearing aid can be unpleasant or even painful, and will certainly be distorted even more. Because of this property of ears and hearing aids, shouting doesn't help someone understand; you may hurt their ears, but that's about all.

You're now aware of what you should not do when dealing with someone with impaired hearing; there are some helpful suggestions about what you *should* do to enhance communication with your hard-of-hearing spouse, parent, or friend. This list is not all-inclusive, but it reflects the feelings of many hearing impaired about what others could do to make life easier for them.

- Speak in a normal tone of voice, or one that is slightly louder than usual. Don't shout. Make an effort to speak clearly and articulate well, but don't exaggerate your mouth and lip movements.
- Try to hold your head still while talking, and don't make extraneous gestures, which can distract attention from the message.
- Be aware that someone with a hearing impairment will be excessively bothered by background noise, so try not to have a television, radio, or other appliance going in the background; understand that hearing may be difficult in a room full of people.
- Don't speak rapidly, but don't slow your speech down to the point where it may seem insulting or downright silly.
- Try and position yourself where the light falls on your face when speaking; don't put your hands near your mouth.
- Because listening is a chore for those with hearing loss, they must take time to rest, especially in a strenuous communication situation such as a party (with multiple speakers and a lot of background noise). If someone wants to be alone for a while, or retreat to a quiet room, accept that decision—don't make an issue of it. People who do this aren't antisocial. They are just tired, and need a break.

Here are some questions commonly asked by family and friends of the hearing impaired:

You say it's important for the light to be on my face so someone can see my mouth. Well, my father has never had lipreading lessons, so why should I bother? Lipreading (more correctly called speechreading, which will be discussed in Chapter 11) is something everyone does, without any special training—although training can make these skills much more efficient. You lipread too, when you're trying to follow a conversation in heavy background noise. See for yourself, the next time you're in such a situation.

Why should I avoid exaggerating my mouth and lip movements? Doesn't it make lipreading easier? On the contrary, it makes it more difficult. Because people aren't used to seeing such movements, they have had no practice reading them.

If people can learn to read lips, why do they still have trouble understanding? The amount of information that can be picked up by reading lips has been greatly overestimated, especially by mystery writers who portray a character who reads lips through binoculars, for example. Perhaps someone with truly exceptional abilities can pick up the thread of a conversation through visual cues alone, but for almost everyone else it is extremely difficult. There are many speech sounds that simply can not be detected visually.

The next chapter will (like the rest of the book) be directed toward those with a hearing loss, but normal-hearing readers who were persuaded to read this chapter might want to continue. Hearing aids, covered in Chapter 6, may be subject to more myth and misunderstanding than any other aspect of hearing impairment.

[6]
The Hearing Aid

This chapter may seem somewhat out of order, coming after a long section on emotional problems and before a discussion of doctors, audiologists, and hearing aid dispensers. However, it is in the middle of the book for a reason. There is a strong temptation to think of a hearing aid as the first step in solving problems associated with a hearing loss. *It is not.* As we've seen in previous chapters, emotional acceptance of the problem, and a willingness to do something about it, comes first.

It is also common to think of a hearing aid as the end process in coping with a hearing loss. That's certainly not true, either. Diligent practice with the aid, hearing therapy, counseling, and a good attitude must go hand-in-hand with wearing the aid.

That's why the discussion of hearing aids is in the middle of the book. Getting a hearing aid is, actually, somewhere in the middle of the process of coping with a hearing loss.

Many of you are wearing a hearing aid now, but are not happy with it. Some of you have never worn an aid, and would like some specific information on the various models and the benefits they offer. Still others may have worn a hearing aid for a while and given up on it. If that's the case, your problems may have stemmed from lack of knowledge about what an aid can and can not do. Let's first consider those benefits and limitations.

A hearing aid can . . .

. . . make soft sound louder, bringing speech to a more comfortable level for listening. Simply because of the increase in loudness, your understanding of speech will probably be improved.

. . . allow you to hear in some situations that used to give you trouble, such as in church. Even though the aid might not enable you to hear every word of a distant speaker, you will pick up more sounds. These sounds will serve as cues to enable you to fill in the parts you miss, possibly through lipreading.

. . . help you to hear high-pitched sounds, such as bird calls. Not only do high-pitched sounds give you more of a "live" feeling (being in touch with the world around you), they also aid in your ability to understand speech.

. . . help you to feel more at ease in social situations, by making it easier for you to understand what's being said. The aid can also alert people to the fact that you don't hear well, and this may induce them to make an extra effort when communicating with you. If you still attach a stigma to hearing loss, this may be hard for you to accept; if so, a simple change in hairstyle will camouflage most aids.

A hearing aid can not . . .

. . . enable you to hear extremely soft sounds. If the hearing aid were set to amplify all the very soft sounds that a normal-hearing person could detect, louder sounds would blast intolerably. Even with a hearing aid that works perfectly, you will still have the equivalent of a mild loss.

. . . cure distortion. The aid only modifies sound going into your ear. If your inner ear and brain distort sound (causing difficulty in *discrimination*, the ability to understand), the hearing aid will help somewhat just by making the sound louder. But even though the sound is louder, the aid can't cure the distortion; it can only make the distorted sound louder and give you a better chance of figuring it out.

. . . restore a completely natural sound. The hearing aid is, after all, an electrical and mechanical device, and therefore will slightly change the quality of what you hear, just as a radio does. Some people describe the sound of a hearing aid as "mechanical" or "tinny." Because it's a relatively small instrument, the aid can not amplify all frequencies; music, for example, will not retain all of its rich harmonics.

. . . allow you to hear well when there is a lot of background noise or many people talking all at once. By adjusting the volume of your aid(s) you may hear better, but these are the situations where the aid will be of least help to you. The aids can not amplify only what you want to hear. You will need to rely on your lipreading again.

. . . amplify only what you want to hear. The aid will also amplify background noise, the sound of your own footsteps, appliance motors running, the sounds of yourself chewing. You probably haven't heard these sounds normally in quite some time, because of the gradual onset of your hearing loss, and it will take some time to adjust to hearing them well again.

To sum up: Hearing aids can not restore normal hearing. They can, however, help you make the most of what hearing you have. You can usually function in a fairly normal way even though you don't hear normally.

How do hearing aids work? An aid is divided into five major parts (shown in Figure 2), all of which play a role in amplifying sound and directing it into your ear. It is important for you to know something about the structure of the aid, because you are likely to have difficulties from time to time, and a working knowledge of the device can help you solve simple problems and save yourself a great deal of frustration.

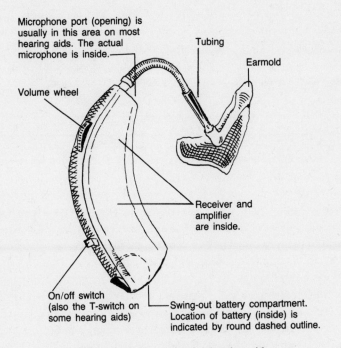

Figure 2. Basic parts of a hearing aid

The *microphone* picks up sound and turns it into electrical energy.

The *battery* provides the power for the aid to work.

The *amplifier*, using the power from the battery, boosts the intensity of the tiny electrical signal from the microphone.

The *receiver* turns the amplified electrical signal back into sound again.

The *earmold* modifies this sound slightly, and directs it into your ear. The earmold, a hollow piece of plasticlike material molded specifically for your ear, extends a half-inch or so into the ear canal; it also helps to hold the aid in place.

In addition to these five basic parts, hearing aids also come equipped with a *volume control* to control the amount of loudness, just like the volume control on a radio. Many aids also have an on-off switch.

Although hearing aids have these same basic components, their appearance may vary quite a bit. Different styles have evolved to suit the preferences of various users. This wide assortment often leaves a newcomer feeling somewhat bewildered. However, once you realize that hearing aids fall into one of *four basic styles*—and learn the advantages and disadvantages of each—things won't seem nearly as confusing. The four basic styles are behind-the-ear, in-the-ear, eyeglass, and body aids. Examples of each type are pictured and described below.

Behind-the-Ear Hearing Aids

Behind-the-ear hearing aids, such as the one shown in Figure 3, are quite popular. Currently, behind-the-ear styles account for about 46 percent of total hearing aid sales.

This type of aid is encased in a plastic compartment about one to one-and-a-half inches long, and a half-inch thick. The aid rests behind the ear, with a piece of flexible tubing going over the top of the ear and connecting the aid to the earmold. The earmold, depending on its type, extends from one quarter to three quarters of an inch into the ear canal.

Advantages. Behind-the-ear styles are popular because they are relatively small and inconspicuous. From the standpoint of an audiologist, behind-the-ear aids are versatile because they can be designed to fit a wide variety of hearing problems. These aids are also easily interchangeable if one has to go in for service.

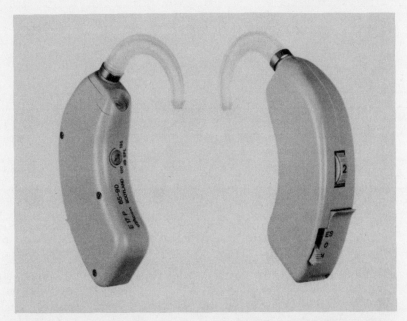

Figure 3. A behind-the-ear aid. This is worn behind the ear with the hook of the aid extending up over the top of the ear and connecting to an earmold.(Photo courtesy of Oticon Corp.)

Disadvantages. In a few cases, people with glasses have difficulty wearing a behind-the-ear aid. If the earpiece of the eyeglasses is exceptionally large, or if the lens prescription is so precise that a slight alteration of position is distracting, a behind-the-ear style may not be advisable. Also, some people just don't have enough space between their ear and the side of their head to accomodate the device.

In-the-Ear Hearing Aids

In-the-ear hearing aids (also called all-in-the-ear), such as the one shown in Figure 4, have gained a great deal of popularity in the past three years or so. About 52 percent of hearing aids now sold are in-the-ear types. To manufacture this aid, an impression is made of the ear canal and the bowl-like opening of the outer ear; the components are then built into a plastic case that is molded from the impression.

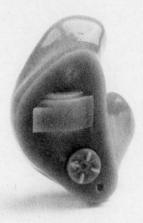

Figure 4. An in-the-ear aid. This fits within the bowl-shaped opening of the outer ear. (Photo courtesy of Oticon Corp.)

Advantages. The in-the-ear aid will not interfere with eyeglasses, and many people feel this type of aid is easier to put on and take off than a behind-the-ear style; it may therefore be helpful to people with arthritis or some other problem with manual dexterity. An in-the-ear aid may also, depending on your hearing loss, provide more power in the high pitches, which can help you understand speech more easily. Don't buy this style of aid only because you think it will be less visible. From a front view, and the side (with most hairstyles), a behind-the-ear style is actually less noticeable.

Disadvantages. Because they are molded individually, you can't try most in-the-ear aids on before you order them. Because the aid fills up your ear, it may be uncomfortable in hot weather. In-the-ear aids are generally reliable, but some people feel they require more repairs than behind-the-ear styles. Repair time poses another problem: If your in-the-ear aid goes in for repair, your loaner will probably be a behind-the-ear model, and you'll need a separate earmold to use it. Most in-the-ear aids are made in one piece. However, one design incorporates a separate case for the workings *and* an earmold that disconnects from the case. This "modular" design means that you can have a new earmold made if the shape or size of your ear canal changes (as sometimes happens), instead of having the whole aid put into a new case, a rather expensive job. Also, the dealer may be able to lend you another modular casing if yours has to be fixed. An earmold for a modular in-the-ear aid won't fit on a behind-the-ear aid, though. The modular design is usually a bit bulkier and more visible.

A recent variation of the in-the-ear style is a canal aid, popularized by President Reagan. This type of aid fits down into the ear with very little protruding into the bowl area of the outer ear. Don't think it's invisible, though. It can easily be seen when someone looks into the ear.

The canal aid has some disadvantages, primarily because of the problems in getting a good fit and the significantly higher cost per aid. Also the size of the wearer's ear canal must be fairly large, the hearing loss can not be very severe, and there must be a hearing loss at all pitches.

This style of aid has only been used since 1982 and may benefit from further research before it can be used on the general population. If you are interested, ask your dispenser if you are a candidate for this particular type of aid.

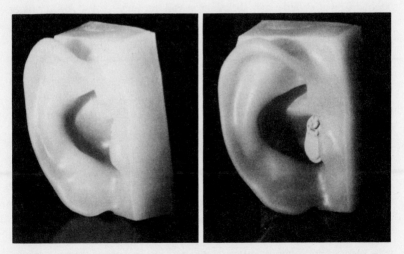

Figure 5. Another in-the-ear style. This is a canal aid. (Photo courtesy of Telex Communications, Inc.)

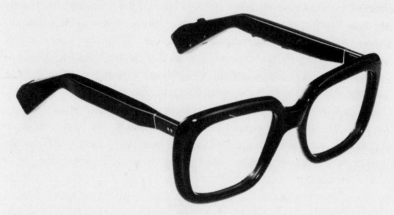

Figure 6. An eyeglass aid. A tube leads from the temple of the eyeglass frame to an earmold. (Photo courtesy of Oticon Corp.)

Eyeglass Hearing Aids

Eyeglass hearing aids have the components built into the temple of the frame. This causes some enlargement of the frame, but with modern technology the parts are so miniaturized that the enlargement of the eyeglasses is hardly noticeable. Eyeglass hearing aids currently account for about 1 percent of total hearing aid sales.

Advantages. Some users feel that any eyeglass aid is less conspicuous than other types; there is, however, a tube that leads from the earpiece of the glasses to the earmold. From a technical standpoint, eyeglass aids allow a procedure called CROS (Contralateral Routing Of Signals) fitting. CROS-fitting means there are two parts of the aid on either ear with a wire running through the bridge of the eyeglasses, connecting those two parts. There are primarily two types of cases appropriate for this fitting. One is a person with a severe hearing loss in only one ear. Sound from a microphone near the bad ear is routed into the good ear.

For technical reasons, this type of fitting is also appropriate for someone who needs amplification in only the high frequencies, not the lows.

(Incidentally, CROS-fitting can also be done with a wire extending across the back of the head between two behind-the-ear aids.)

Disadvantages. There are many. First of all, fitting is difficult. You must buy a new set of frames, possibly lenses also, and run back and forth between the hearing aid dispenser and the optician, trying to get everything adjusted. Eyeglass aids need more repair than other styles, which brings up another drawback: When either the aid or the glasses need repair, you're out both—unless you happen to have an extra set of glasses, an extra hearing aid, or both. It can also be a nuisance to constantly have your eyes and ears connected. There may be many times when you want to wear only your glasses and not fuss with the hearing aid, such as when you shave or exercise.

Body Aids

Body aids, such as the one shown in Figure 7, are about half the size of a cigarette pack, and are usually worn on the chest. A cord leads from the box to a buttonlike device that connects to the earmold. Less than 1 percent of aids sold are of this type, and are usually prescribed for young children.

Advantages. In cases of near-total deafness, where a tremendous amount of power is needed, only the body aid can provide it. Also, people who have physical disabilities that make it hard for them to handle a smaller device often benefit from a body aid.

Disadvantages. A body aid is more visible and rather cumbersome. It is not used very often in cases of age-related hearing loss.

With all these types of aids to choose from, you should have little trouble finding one that suits your individual needs and preferences. The technology, by the way, is truly marvelous. The hearing aid industry has advanced more in the last ten years than during the previous thirty, when the modern hearing aid was being developed. Much of this advancement is due to the space program. The search for ways to miniaturize equipment in a space capsule has paid off in many ways, including compact and reliable hearing aids, heart pacemakers implanted in the chest, and the familiar pocket calculator.

There's another effect of these recent technological breakthroughs:

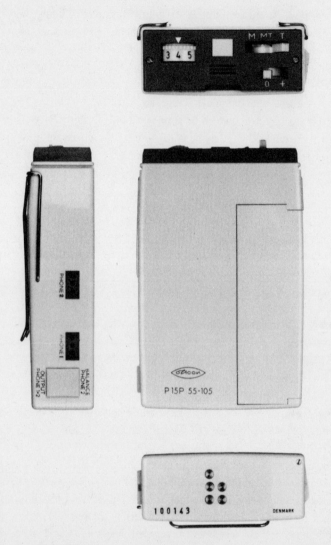

Figure 7. A body aid. This is worn on the body with a cord leading up to an earmold. (Photo courtesy of Oticon Corp.)

Hearing aid users are now buying new aids on the average of one every three years because they want to take advantage of more modern, increasingly sophisticated models. A hearing aid certainly can be expected to last longer than three years, but eventually will wear out and have to be replaced.

Why? Because hearing aids are extremely delicate pieces of equipment, and get pretty rough handling. On top of this, consumers demand that aids be small—which makes them less durable—and relatively inexpensive. Manufacturers probably could build a hearing aid that would last a lifetime, but it would be prohibitively expensive (not that an aid is cheap, now; costs will be discussed more fully in Chapter 9).

With reasonable care, a hearing aid can last five years or so; longer if you're meticulous about proper handling, care, and maintenance. Here are some suggestions on how to preserve what is, after all, a substantial investment:

- Be careful of moisture. Keep the aid away from steamy kitchens, or bathrooms where someone has just taken a hot shower. Also, be careful not to hit the aid with hair spray, or other aerosols. Getting caught in the rain won't do your hearing aid any good, but droplets of water aren't as harmful as vapor. Usually, your hair or a hat will keep rain water from harming the aid. Never wear the aid while bathing.
- Don't expose the aid to intense heat. Leaving it on the window sill in bright sushine can damage it, as might setting the aid on top of a radiator.
- Protect it from shock. Don't handle the aid roughly, and never set it where it could be knocked to the floor.
- Protect it from dust. Small dust particles can clog up the openings to the microphone. Remove the aid when you are in dusty environments.
- The earmold or the canal opening of the in-the-ear aid may sometimes get wax lodged in the small holes in the part that goes down into the ear. If the wax is near the edge of the hole, carefully pick the wax out with a pin or toothpick, being careful not to damage the opening.

If the wax has worked its way farther into the opening of an earmold you can clean this yourself. Disconnect the earmold and the flexible tubing from the hearing aid itself. Just carefully pull apart— you won't break anything. *Don't* pull the earmold and the tubing apart; they are glued together. Now that the earmold and tubing are disconnected from the aid, soak them overnight in warm water. (*Never* use hot water because you will melt the glue that bonds them.) In the morning, rinse the earmold and connecting tube with clean water, dry them thoroughly, and fit them back on the aid.

If wax becomes lodged farther into the opening of an in-the-ear aid, you must see your hearing aid dispenser for professional cleaning.

• Once a year, have the aid cleaned and checked by your dealer or dispenser (there's a distinction, which will be explained in Chapter 9, but both terms refer to the person who sold you the aid).

An aid probably will need repair from time to time—but you can cut your trips to the dispenser by doing your troubleshooting. Often the problem is minor. This troubleshooting chart will help you recognize and correct some of the more common simple problems.

Hearing Aid Troubleshooting

Problem	What to do
Aid does not work at all	Try a new battery. (The precedure for inserting a battery should have been explained by the person who sold you the aid. If not, get an explanation now, or check the instructions that came with the aid.)
	Check to make sure that the battery is not reversed (with the plus and minus sides facing in the wrong directions).
	Inspect the tubing to insure that it is not bent and crimping off the sound.
	Make certain that the earmold is not plugged with wax.
	If the hearing aid has a T-switch for telephone use (more on this in Chapter 10) make sure it is not in the T position.
	Still not working? Call the dispenser.
Aid is working, but weak	Replace the battery. Batteries give full output until the last few hours of life. As soon as the battery starts to weaken, throw it away.
	Make sure that the earmold is inserted properly.
	Your ear canal may be plugged with wax. A doctor can easily check it out.

Problem

What to do

Aid gives intermittent or scratchy signal

The on-off switch may be dusty where it makes electrical contact inside the aid. Turn the switch on and off several times.

If it's a body aid, check the cords for crimping or fraying.

If it still gives an intermittent or scratchy signal, the aid needs repair.

Aid makes whistling or squealing sound

The hearing aid is feeding back, just as a loudspeaker feeds back if a microphone is too close: The sound of the loudspeaker is picked up by the microphone, amplified by the speaker, picked up again by the microphone, amplified again, and so on—until the sound has been amplified to a loud howl. To find out why your hearing aid is feeding back, first take the aid off and cover up any opening in the earmold (including the tiny vent holes that are sometimes drilled) and see if the feedback stops. If it *does* stop, the earmold may not have been correctly inserted, or else it does not fit your ear properly. See your dispenser for instructions again on how to insert it properly, or for another earmold.

If it still squeals, take off the tubing and earmold. Place your finger over the end of the hearing aid that the tubing fits on (the hook). If the squealing stops, the tubing is probably cracked, or does not fit properly into the earmold. See your dispenser for repair.

If the squealing continues, there is probably some internal damage, and the aid needs repair.

Aid uses up batteries too quickly

Battery life is determined by the power of the aid and the type of battery, and can be anywhere from 50 to 1,000 hours of *use*—when the hearing aid is actually on. The average battery life is probably close to 150 hours. The hearing aid dispenser can give you an estimate of battery life based on your particular aid and the brand of batteries you use. You should keep a diary

Problem   **What to do**

of the number of hours the aid is in use; the time may be much longer than you realize.

Maybe you are buying too many batteries at a time or from a place that keeps them on the shelf for a long time. (The term "shelf life" is used to refer to battery life. After several months, batteries begin to gradually lose power even if they are still in the package.) One package, usually about six batteries, should last a reasonable amount of time.

If you still feel the batteries are being used up too quickly, check to see if you may accidently be leaving the aid turned on at night.

Are batteries still draining too quickly? There may be an electronic problem, so take the aid in for repair.

Moisture
collects in
the tubing
of the aid

This is common. As the warm air from the inside of your ear goes into the cooler tubing the water vapor will condense and collect on the tubing. This will usually not cause a problem unless there is a great deal of moisture, in which case the tubing can become plugged. You can buy a small dehumidifier pack from your dealer to store your aid in at night. This will reduce the moisture, but you'll have to have the tubing changed more frequently because it will dry out sooner.

Difficulties with hearing aids don't always, of course, stem from trouble with the instrument itself. The new experience of wearing an aid can be difficult to cope with. There may be no simple solution; however, an understanding of why the situation annoys you may help you to deal with the problem. Here are some of the more common difficulties:

Hearing Aid User Complaints

Problem	Explanation
When I work in the kitchen, the sound of dishes clinking together drives me crazy.	You are bothered by sudden high-frequency sounds, such as dishes clinking. It is probably quite annoying because you haven't heard these sounds in a while, or you have only heard the low frequencies in these sounds. In some cases, a condition called *recruitment* (an abnormal sensitivity to loudness) will cause sudden, high-frequency sounds to be uncomfortable. You may soon adjust to the new sounds coming through the hearing aid, though. If you can't get used to them, the hearing aid dispenser may adjust the aid.
I hate the unnatural sound of the hearing aid.	Since you have a hearing loss, "natural" for you means not hearing well. As mentioned earlier in the chapter, the hearing aid must change the nature of sound; the change, while less natural-sounding, will allow better hearing. Most hearing aid users become accustomed to this different type of sound.
I get so much wax in my ears, now that I wear a hearing aid.	The presence of the earmold may stimulate wax production. People who don't wear hearing aids get wax in their ears, too, but it gradually falls out of the ear canal. With an earmold in place, much of the wax is retained. You may have to visit a physician from time to time and have the wax removed; this is a simple and painless procedure.
The earmold hurts.	In the beginning, the earmold will be slightly uncomfortable. It's much like wearing a new pair of shoes, and you will probably soon become used to it. However, if the earmold still is uncomfortable after a few days, or if you notice irritated spots in your ear, go back to the dispenser and have the earmold altered.

Problem

Everything
is so loud!
I can't stand it.

Explanation

When you're coming out of a movie theater into bright sunshine, the light hurts your eyes. Much the same situation occurs when you have become used to a hearing loss and suddenly put on an aid. It may take days or weeks for you to adjust to your new-found hearing when you first get an aid. If you still are bothered after three of four weeks, or if it is actually painful to wear the aid at any time, return to the dispenser. Having the characteristics of the aid readjusted may allow a compromise between good hearing and tolerance of the sound.

I wore my new
hearing aid to a
meeting yesterday
and it was
unbearable.

A hearing aid takes getting used to, and a room full of people is not the place to start. Begin by wearing the aid alone in a quiet room, and read aloud. After you've become used to the sound of your own voice, invite another person in to speak with you. Gradually increase the number of people in the communication situation; you may also want to experiment with various levels of background noise to simulate real-world conditions. Putting on the aid and immediately venturing into a difficult communication situation can quickly alienate a new wearer; this is one reason why so many aids wind up in the drawer after only one use. You will probably want to allow three or four weeks before you are wearing the aid full time in all types of situations.

My own voice
sounds strange.

This is normal because you are not used to hearing yourself as others hear you. Remember the first time you heard yourself on a tape recorder? You will adjust to the "new voice" within a few days. But if your voice continues to sound hollow or it echoes (or you have a "full" feeling in your ear) report this problem to your hearing

Problem   **Explanation**

aid dispenser, who can adjust the aid and/or your earmold.

If you've never worn a hearing aid, and are considering getting one, knowing about these typical problems beforehand will, at least, let you know that you're not alone. *All* the problems haven't been covered, of course; it's evident—just from the length of this chapter—how broad the topic is. Related information will be presented in later chapters: how an audiologist (Chapter 8) selects the right kind of hearing aid, and how to deal with the people who sell hearing aids (Chapter 9). You should see a physician before getting an aid, and that will be the subject of the next chapter. First, here are some of the more common questions asked about hearing aids:

What brand of hearing aid should I buy? You are best off if you stick to a major brand, but no one brand is best for everybody. It is not the brand, but the particular model, that is important. Different types of hearing losses require various hearing aid models; if a particular brand is recommended to you it is probably because that manufacturer makes a model with characteristics that fit your hearing loss. But it does not mean that the particular manufacturer is the *only* one who makes the right type of aid. A listing of major hearing aid brands is included in Chapter 9.

I know that you have used "style" to describe the way a hearing aid is worn, that is, behind-the-ear, in-the-ear, and so on. And I know what "brand" means. But then what do you mean by "model"? Model refers to the characteristics that are built into a hearing aid, determining the quantity and quality of sound that the hearing aid can provide. As noted above, different types of hearing losses require different combinations of these characteristics. Each particular combination that a manufacturer makes is called a model. A large hearing aid manufacturer, for example, might make twenty different models of behind-the-ear aids, each of which is designed to fit the needs of a particular hearing loss.

The four major characteristics are:

1. *Gain*—the power of the instrument, how much it amplifies sound. The greater your hearing loss, the more gain you'll probably need.

2. *Frequency range*—how much power there is in certain pitch ranges, and how far the amplification ability of the aid extends into the high and low pitches. If, for example, you have a loss in the high frequencies (perhaps because of many years of exposure to loud noise) you will need an aid designed to boost high frequencies.

3. *Maximum power output*—the loudest sound the aid will produce, regardless of how much sound is put into it. This characteristic insures comfort, and acts as a safeguard against damage to the ears.

4. *Distortion*—a measure of how faithfully the hearing aid reproduces the sound that comes into it. Any electronic instrument, including your television, for example, distorts the sound signal to some extent, which is why you may have trouble understanding actors and speakers. There is a triple distortion: the television, your impaired hearing mechanism, and the hearing aid itself. On top of all that, you really can't read lips on television, and it's hard to pick up other cues that would help you to understand.

I notice many of my friends wearing two hearing aids. Why is that? Good question. There are many advantages to wearing binaural (two) aids, and the practice has recently become much more popular. Although wearing two aids can be more bothersome and will be more expensive, you'll benefit from not having a "bad side." You will feel more oriented or balanced in space with two aids. Having two ears to listen with helps you to localize sound much more easily, so you'll spend less time spinning your head around, trying to figure out who is talking to you among a group of people; this is extremely helpful if you are lipreading, and need to pick up on conversation quickly. There's another advantage, too: Background noise can be less troublesome when you are listening with two ears. Have a friend with normal hearing try this experiment to prove it: Plug one ear tightly and carry on a conversation while there is quite a bit of background noise. The noise will seem much more distracting when the ear is plugged. Another advantage to wearing two aids is that neither of the aids has to be turned up as loudly as when wearing only one. This helps in background noise and in overall comfort. But probably the biggest advantage to wearing two aids is that you will hear better. There is more information going to your brain so it is easier to figure out the message.

Keep in mind that not everyone will benefit from binaural aids, though. A person who has a large difference in the hearing loss between ears probably won't be helped at all. The ear with the more severe hearing loss usually also has more severe discrimination problems. A hearing aid in that ear would produce loud, distorted sound that might actually interfere with the clearer sound in the better ear. An audiologist will be able to determine if two aids are right for you. By the way, two aids won't cost double the price of one. The reason will be explained in Chapter 9.

Do I have to wear the hearing aid all the time? For the first few weeks you may want to wear the aid at least six to eight hours a day to practice using it in different situations. After you develop good judgment about the benefits of the aid, you can wear it whenever you think you need to. You'll probably want to wear it most of the time, anyway.

I feel embarrassed about wearing the aid. When will I get over it? Probably as soon as you fully realize all the benefits of wearing the aid. For some people, embarrassment is a natural reaction, but remember that a hearing aid is much less visible than you probably think it is. Besides, by wearing the aid you can save yourself a lot of embarrassment that stems from mistakes in conversation.

I don't have a hearing aid at the present time. How do I tell when I really need one? You need an aid when you are having significant difficulty in communication, and a physician has told you that there is no medical help. If you are not hearing things that you need to or want to, you are probably a good candidate. An audiologist can confirm your suspicions, but can not tell whether you are having problems—only you can tell that for sure. Don't be satisfied with just "getting along OK." It is much better to be "doing well." Different people in different situations will vary in their need for a hearing aid. A retired person who lives alone will have very different needs than a librarian, who constantly deals with people who are speaking softly.

Where do I buy batteries for a hearing aid? What kind do I buy? Buy batteries at the same place you bought the hearing aid. Drug stores often carry them, but since the demand is not so high, the batteries are less likely to be fresh. By the same token, don't buy batteries too far ahead, as their shelf life is about six months. One package usually holds about six batteries. As mentioned previously, it's a good idea to keep track of battery life—just like checking mileage on a car—so you'll be able to tell if a battery is exhausted unusually quickly. As far as the type of batteries to buy, follow the recommendation of the dispenser for the right battery to power your aid. Mercury batteries have slightly less power than silver oxide batteries, but last longer and are less expensive. The zinc/air battery has just recently been introduced; it has about the same power as a mercury battery, but lasts twice as long and costs twice as much. You won't save money, but you will spend less time changing batteries.

Is there any hearing aid that does not have anything that goes inside the ear? Yes, there is; it's called a bone conduction aid and was used in the past for people who had a conductive hearing loss. The aid was really a vibrator on a headband, usually worn against the bone in back of the ear. This system vibrated the bones of the skull, bypassed the inadequate outer or middle ear, and sent the sound directly to the inner ear (which would, for this application, be normal).

These aids are bulky, uncomfortable at times, and do not provide a very clear sound. They are rarely used today because the other types of aids, described previously, are better.

[7]
The Physician

Once you've made the decision to get a hearing aid, you must eventually be seen by a physician. In fact, according to a regulation of the Food and Drug Administration, the hearing aid dispenser is not supposed to sell you a hearing aid until you have done so. Before you buy the aid, you must produce a note from the doctor, certifying that there is no medical reason why you should not have a hearing aid. There are several good reasons for this:

- Before the federal regulation concerning the visit to the doctor, some people were being sold hearing aids when there was a medical or surgical technique that could restore some or all of their hearing.
- In unusual cases, a hearing loss can be the symptom of a serious medical problem. For example, a hearing loss can be caused by diabetes, a thyroid condition, or a tumor on the auditory nerve.
- There are certain medical conditions that can be aggravated by a hearing aid, such as an ear infection.

A physician who specializes in diseases of the ear should be able to spot any of these situations, although the clearance you need can be obtained from any type of medical doctor. The regulation was written this way because specialists are hard to find in some remote areas of the country. However, you should visit a specialist if at all possible.

The kind of doctor you want to see is usually called an ear, nose, and throat doctor, or ENT. An ENT is a physician who has earned a medical degree and then undertaken extra study in the ear, nose, and throat field, combined with a residency at a hospital. ENT physicians are also known as head and neck surgeons or as *otorhinolaryngologists* (*oto* means ear, *rhino* indicates nose, and *laryngo* stands for throat). ENT means the same thing, and is a lot easier to say. Some of these specialists limit their practice entirely to ears and call themselves *otologists*.

Does this mean that an ENT or otologist will be an expert on hearing aids and other aspects of coping with hearing loss? No, it does not: While these physicians are highly trained in the pathology of the ear, and possess great skill in medical and surgical procedures, they may not be well versed in the problems caused by a communication handicap and the rehabilitative procedures available. Some ENTs take a personal interest in communication problems, but with the staggering amount of research they must keep up with, it's next to impossible for these specialists to be aware of all the developments in the field of *aural rehabilitation* (therapy to help a hearing-impaired person communicate better).

This essentially means that it will be your responsibility to make sure you're getting an informed opinion on the topic of hearing aids and communication problems. Don't be afraid to question your doctor, to discuss your communication problems, or to ask for a referral to someone who might be more adept in these matters. First, though, be satisfied that there is nothing that can be done medically or surgically to alleviate your hearing loss.

If, for example, you suffer from otosclerosis (where the tiny sound-conducting bones in the middle ear lose their ability to vibrate), surgery may help to restore hearing. Also, most hearing losses that result from middle ear infections can be treated medically or surgically. A general rule of thumb states that if the problem is centered in the outer or middle ear, there's a chance that it may be cured. If the loss is secondary to another condition such as poor circulation, an infection, a metabolic imbalance, or a tumor, medical treatment is indicated for the primary problem.

Inner-ear hearing losses rarely respond to any sort of treatment, however. The damage from noise exposure or normal deterioration is irreversible. If the hearing loss results from deterioration of nerve pathways up to the brain, it's permanent. *Only a physician can tell for sure if medical or surgical intervention can help your particular case.*

A fairly new development in the area of help for the hearing-impaired is the cochlear implant. In this expensive major surgical procedure, an electrode is inserted into the inner ear (cochlea). After the surgery has healed, the person wears a small electronic device on the upper body that analyzes sound picked up by a microphone near the ear. The resulting signal is sent to the electrode in the inner ear, which directly stimulates the auditory nerve.

The media have done a great job of publicizing this new technique, even called it a "bionic ear." What they do not tell you is, first of all, that the surgery may destroy the inner ear, so that only people who are totally deaf and have nothing to lose are selected for the surgery, which is done in only a few places around the country.

A second very important fact is that the procedure does not bring back the ability to understand speech. What is "heard" by these patients is only a very distorted awareness of sounds in their environment. They can not recognize most of the sounds and certainly can not understand speech through the implant alone. What the device does do is put the person back in touch with an "auditory world" and provide enough information through the ear to help a great deal in the lipreading process.

There is ongoing research where several electrodes are placed in the inner ear, and the results claim to provide a clearer signal. However, it will be many years before the procedure has advanced to the point where people without total losses will benefit or where those with the implant will be able to follow conversation without a great deal of lipreading.

What will happen when you visit the doctor for the medical examination that is needed before you can buy a hearing aid? First, the doctor will probably take an extensive case history of your problem, and then look in your ears with an *otoscope*, the familiar flashlight device found in most doctors' offices. The ENT will be looking for any obvious problem with the ear canal or eardrum.

The next step may involve tests for balance and coordination; these are done to see if the hearing loss might stem from a neurological problem. The doctor may also use a tuning fork to make a rough estimate of how well you can hear the sound it gives off.

Following the examination, the doctor may recommend an evaluation by an audiologist (next chapter) or other tests, depending on what was found during the examination. Often, you may be asked to return after these tests are carried out. ENTs sometimes have an audiologist on staff who may do the hearing test during your visit. In either case, there will be an extra charge for the test.

Eventually, the doctor will give you a diagnosis and recommendations; this is when problems can arise. Doctors may be in a hurry and anxious to move on to other scheduled patients. As a result, they sometimes give instructions rather than explanations. It is very important that you ask questions at this point and insist on a complete explanation of your problem. If you don't understand, ask the doctor to restate it in simpler terms. What the doctor says will be very important to you, and since you are paying for it, *you have a right to a thorough explanation, as well as a discussion of all your alternatives.*

Here are some questions you might want to ask. If you think you may get flustered and forget, take this list with you.

Questions to Ask Your Doctor

- Is there anything that can be done to alleviate my hearing loss?
- Will it be permanent?
- Is there something that can be done medically or surgically? If there is, will I have a residual hearing loss after treatment?
- If surgery is recommended: Is it necessary for my health? Can I get along without surgery? (Some people have hearing loss that could be corrected surgically, but—for their own reasons—choose not to have surgery, and wear a hearing aid. This is all right unless the condition causing the hearing loss endangers health.)
- Can you refer me to a good audiologist, one who is particularly interested in hearing aids and aural rehabilitation? (Some audiologists are more interested in other aspects of hearing loss, such as diagnosis of particular disorders, educational audiology for children, or academic research.)
- How much will all this cost me? How much is the office visit? The hearing test? Any further treatment or tests? (Don't feel as though you're being stingy, by the way. Remember that the richest people in the world got that way because they were careful about how they spent their money.)
- What part of my treatment, if any, is covered by Medicare, Medicaid, or other insurance? (More on this in Chapter 14.)
- Do you think I might benefit from a hearing aid? If not, why?

There may be times when you want a second opinion—especially if surgery is indicated. Admittedly, it's a bother and an additional expense to see another doctor, but you must weigh that against the cost and risk of surgery. Even if no surgery or medical treatment is recommended, you may feel as though your doctor doesn't know or care about your particular problem. Don't ever feel bad about getting a second opinion. Doctors are fallible, and don't have all the answers.

The next chapter will explain the procedures used by audiologists. First, questions on dealing with physicians:

What right do I have to disagree with my doctor? I don't have a medical degree. If you disagree about whether your hearing loss causes a communication problem, you have every right in the world to differ with your doctor. After all, it is your problem, and in that sense you know more about it than anyone else in the world.

Are any of the doctor's tests painful? Not really. The only discomfort you may feel would result from a specialized test called electronystagmography, which often makes people dizzy and nauseated. This test is only done in cases where certain inner-ear problems are suspected.

Doctors are so expensive. Is there any way I can save money? If a hearing loss is your only concern, you can check to see if you really do have a significant hearing loss before you see a doctor. In many places, hearing screenings are offered free or at reduced cost. Check at colleges, health fairs, or senior citizen centers. The result of the hearing test will tell you whether to pursue the matter and see a doctor.

Suppose I want a hearing aid but don't want to see a doctor? The federal regulation allows you to sign a waiver if it is against your personal beliefs to see a doctor; the waiver states that even though you understand it is in your best interest to see a physician, you choose not to. For reasons already explained, using this waiver is not a good idea. Some people who have had hearing aids in the past choose not to see the doctor again (you need clearance every time you buy another aid) but you should be aware that medical problems can develop within this time.

What role do diet and health play in hearing loss? Aging, infection, and noise are not the only cause of acquired hearing losses. Just as with other body organs, the ear can be affected by overall body health. Excessive intake of refined sugar, salt, alcohol, tobacco, and caffeine can cause metabolic imbalances that inhibit body function, including hearing.

Meniere's disease, where there is too much inner-ear fluid, is thought to be linked to metabolic problems. Some people find relief from the symptoms through decreasing sodium and increasing potassium in their diet.

Some people have specific food allergies that lead to pancreatic insufficiencies and thus disorders throughout the body, including the ears.

[8]
The Audiologist

It's odd that even though the number of audiologists in the United States is constantly on the increase, many people have little if any idea of what an audiologist is. Because audiologists are your first line of defense in preventing a hearing loss from making your life difficult and souring your emotional outlook, it is important that you understand what audiologists are, what they can do, and how they do it.

An audiologist is a professional trained in the nonmedical aspects of hearing impairment, such as evaluation of hearing loss and rehabilitation of the hearing impaired.

Audiologists have earned either a master's degree or doctorate, have served an internship, and have passed a qualifying examination. They are certified by the American Speech-Language-Hearing Association, or licensed by the state in which they practice, or both.

Along the way, an audiologist learns how speech and hearing develop; how problems arise with hearing; how various methods of rehabilitation help people with a hearing loss. This type of rehabilitation is called *aural rehabilitation*, and the basic tools are therapy, counseling, and hearing aids.

Although not all audiologists specialize in the same aspect of hearing loss, they generally provide these services:

- A *screening*, to determine if someone has a hearing loss significant enough to follow up on.
- A *hearing evaluation*, a complete set of tests to determine the amount of hearing loss and the degree of handicap that may result.
- A *hearing aid evaluation*, to determine what kind of hearing aid will best suit an individual's hearing loss. In some cases the audiologist will sell hearing aids. Audiologists who have joined this recent trend perfer to call themselves "dispensers" rather than "dealers," a distinction that will be explained in the next chapter.

• *Therapy and counseling*, to help the hearing-impaired person improve communication and cope with the hearing loss. This is a rapidly growing area of audiology, and will be covered in Chapter 11.

Where do you find an audiologist? They usually work in a speech and hearing center, a hospital, an ENT's office, a college or university, or in private practice. They are often listed in the yellow pages. If a college or university in your area trains students in speech and hearing, there is probably a clinic on campus that offers reduced fees because it serves as a training ground for students (who are under the supervision of a fully qualified audiologist).

When calling a college or university, don't ask the person at the switchboard "whether the college gives hearing tests." Switchboard operators may not be completely informed about activities on campus. Instead, ask for the department of *communication disorders, speech and hearing,* or *speech pathology and audiology.* If the operator can't find the first one you ask for, try all three, because the person on the other end of the telephone will probably just be scanning an alphabetical directory, and might not realize that you want *speech pathology and audiology* when you've asked for *speech and hearing.*

Once you are connected with the right department, ask to speak to a faculty member, preferably an audiologist, who should be able to tell you about the availability of hearing tests. Don't ask a secretary or clerk; in large universities, clerical staffers are rotated frequently and you may be speaking to a newcomer who may not know about all of the department's activities.

When you arrange a hearing test at any of the facilities mentioned above you will be given an appointment. If you're confronted with a long waiting time (longer than two weeks or so), you might elect to try another audiologist.

What will the hearing test be like? You will enter a sound-treated booth—a room specially designed to keep out background noise—and will sit facing a window. The audiologist will be on the other side of the window during the testing. First, though, the audiologist will join you in the room and take a case history. If you can not hear or understand the questions, it is essential that you say so. Don't guess and risk giving inappropriate or incomplete answers; the audiologist won't mind a bit if you ask to have words repeated, or spoken more slowly. After all, if you didn't have trouble hearing, you wouldn't be there in the first place.

Following the case history, the audiologist may look in your ears with an otoscope to make sure that there is no obstruction or infection to affect the test results. Then, a pair of headphones will be placed over your ears, and the door to the booth will be shut (but not locked). The audiologist will be at the other side of the window. There will be a microphone channel open, and the audiologist will be able to see and hear you at all times.

Only one test, a *pure tone air conduction test*, is given for a basic screening. Several different tests are given during a hearing evaluation. In each case, you will be given instructions in advance, and although there's really no compelling reason for you to know the purpose of these tests, a description of what will happen may satisfy your curiosity about all the mysterious beeps, soft voices, and other sounds you will hear during the thirty minutes to an hour you spend in a hearing evaluation. Here's what the tests are called, and what they measure:

1. *Pure tone air conduction.* This is the basic sensitivity test, used in both a complete evaluation and a screening (you will probably get only a screening if you are tested at a senior citizen center or health fair. Keep in mind that a very mild hearing loss usually can't be detected at an event such as a health fair, where there is a lot of background noise; under those circumstances, the listener just can't detect quiet sounds). During the pure tone air conduction test, a series of tones, like musical notes, will be fed through the headphones. The test will be done on one ear at a time. The audiologist will ask you to respond whenever you hear the tone, either by raising your hand or pushing a button. You should respond even when the tone is very faint. The tones will be given at all different loudnesses and pitches; the purpose of this test is to determine the softest level at which you can hear in all the frequency ranges. If you remember the material in Chapter 1, you'll understand that this is a test for *sensitivity*. Also, remember that hearing losses occur at different frequencies, so it is important for the audiologist to determine at which frequencies, or pitches, you hear best.

2. *Pure tone bone conduction.* The headphones will be removed for this test. The audiologist will instead place a tiny vibrator behind an ear

or on the forehead. This test proceeds in the same manner as the first test, except that the vibrator bypasses the outer and middle ear and directly measures the sensitivity of the inner ear mechanism.

3. *Speech reception, or speech recognition, threshold testing.* The headphones will be placed back over your ears and the audiologist, through a microphone, will read a list of two-syllable words, such as *baseball, cowboy,* and *railroad.* You are to repeat what was said— there is a microphone in your chamber—or what you think was said. The words will become progressively fainter, and it is important that you take your best guess if you aren't sure of the word spoken. This is part of the test. This test will identify how sensitive your ears are to speech.

4. *Speech discrimination, or word recognition, testing.* This will measure your ability to understand speech once it's loud enough for you. The audiologist will determine an adequate and comfortable level of loudness, and read a list of about fifty one-syllable words for each ear. (Sometimes the audiologist will play a tape of someone else reading the words.) You will be asked, for example, to "say the word *fail.*" The words can be very difficult to recognize—you might mistake *fail* for *sail*—so don't become frustrated. You are expected to make some mistakes.

These tests are not always given in this order, and the word recognition test has several variations. You may also, at any time during these tests, hear a sound like a waterfall in the ear that is not being tested. This noise blocks out that ear to make sure that you're not picking up sound where you are not supposed to.

There are some other tests which may be given. *Impedance*, a test of middle ear function, involves bouncing a sound wave off the eardrum and analyzing the return wave. In this procedure, the audiologist does all the work. All you have to do is let the audiologist rather firmly insert an earplug, which may be slightly uncomfortable, but certainly not painful. You will then feel some pressure changes and hear some loud sounds.

Following the hearing evaluation, the audiologist will discuss whether or not a hearing aid is appropriate. If a hearing aid is indicated, another appointment will be set up for a *hearing aid evaluation*, where further tests will determine what model aid is best for you. The audiologist may take an impression for a custom-made earmold for you to be used in the hearing aid evaluation. In the meantime it is a good idea to see an ENT physician (if you have not already seen one) to make sure that there is no medical problem, and to receive the clearance you will need to eventually purchase an aid. If you have transportation problems, the audiologist may elect to do the hearing aid evaluation immediately, but that is the exception and not the rule.

After the hearing aid evaluation, the audiologist will recommend the type of aid you should buy; a dispensing audiologist can sell you the aid, although you're under no obligation to buy it from the person who does the hearing aid evaluation. In most cases, the audiologist will refer you to people who sell aids.

How is the right type of aid determined? There's no general consensus about the best way to go about it, but most audiologists use one or more variations of the following procedures:

- The audiologist will ask the client to make judgments on what is the most comfortable level of loudness, and also the level at which loudness becomes uncomfortable. On the basis of this, and the results of previous tests, appropriate general characteristics are determined. Aids with these general characteristics are chosen from a stock, and each is tried on the client for comparison during various tests. These tests, which are done through loudspeakers instead of earphones, gauge ability to hear tones and/or understand speech.

- Sometimes the audiologist will judge the necessary characteristics from the results of the hearing test and will use mathematical formulas to recommend the right aid. A few audiologists don't keep a stock of aids for the clients to try out; it is sometimes felt that since the client may not be using a personalized earmold during the testing of the aids, the results won't be all that meaningful. Another school of thought holds that once the general characteristics are established, there's really no significant difference among the various makes of hearing aid.

Depending on the audiologist's philosophy and judgment, the final recommendation may be *generic*—just a recommendation of the characteristics of the kind of aid you need. Or, the audiologist might suggest a specific brand name and model, even a serial number. Why? Because if a special characteristic is needed, there may be only one company that manufactures a model suitable. There are other reasons why an audiologist may choose to recommend a specific brand: Experience may have shown that it has better repair services, or may be more convenient because of greater adjustability.

Those audiologists who are not dispensers will give you a list of hearing aid dealers in town who they feel are competent and ethical. Even if the audiologist is a dispenser, you may request this list if you choose to buy elsewhere. When you discuss these matters with your audiologist, keep in mind that it is perfectly all right for you to:

- Ask if there is a specific dispenser on the list who is most appropriate for your needs.
- Shop around among those on the list.
- Ask for a general idea of what costs will be and what services should be included.

You should also be given the opportunity to discuss different styles of hearing aids (behind-the-ear, in-the-ear, etc.) with the audiologist. The advantages and disadvantages of each, as they relate to your personal needs, should be considered. If the audiologist feels that one style is particularly appropriate, you should ask for the reasons why.

You're now ready to go out and purchase an aid, the topic of the next chapter. First, let's consider some of the more frequently asked questions about audiologists, hearing tests, and hearing aid recommendations:

How much does an audiologist charge? The prices will vary widely, but you can probably expect to pay from $25 to $75 for a hearing evaluation, and $40 to $80 for a hearing aid evaluation. Prices will be lower at a college or university clinic.

If I go to a clinic at a college or university, won't I be taking a chance by letting students test me? Students in these clinics are under the direct supervision of a fully qualified (and at many institutions, exceptionally qualified) audiologist. As a matter of fact, the audiologists responsible for the students may be paying closer attention to the tests than if they were doing them themselves. All results and recommendations will, of course, be reviewed by the supervising audiologist. There is one drawback:

Students need more time to conduct the tests, and you occasionally may have to sit around and wait a while, when something is being explained to them. But because the cost will be lower than if you were tested in a hospital or at a private practice, it may be worth it to you.

The audiologist I'm seeing is called Dr. Robinson. Audiologists aren't doctors, are they? They are not medical doctors, but some audiologists—usually those in private practice or at universities—have a doctorate in audiology. This degree is earned after about three to five years of additional study beyond the master's degree.

How do the results of my tests get to my doctor and hearing aid dispenser? Part of the audiologist's service involves writing reports and forwarding them to your doctor. You can request a copy of the report if you like, although it is written in technical language and may be hard to understand. The information about the kind of hearing aid you need will usually be given to you, since you are likely to contact several dispensers.

[9]
The Hearing Aid Dispenser

You've probably been wondering when this book would get around to explaining the distinction between a hearing aid "dispenser" and a hearing aid "dealer." The terms have been used interchangeably so far, and you may be somewhat confused—but since the terms actually have no strict definition, it's hard to say when one or the other is correct.

Both refer to someone who sells hearing aids. The primary difference between a hearing aid dispenser and a hearing aid dealer is basically the same as the difference between a *trailer* and a *mobile home,* or an *undertaker* and a *funeral director.* One phrase sounds better than the other, you see, and people concerned with their image have a way of working a more impressive-sounding word into their vocabulary.

When audiologists began to sell hearing aids, they decided that the term *dealer* didn't sound professional enough, and the term *dispenser* was popularized. Recently, the dealers began to express a marked preference toward being called dispensers, too.

Before audiologists moved into the market, hearing aids were sold by members of the commercial establishment who usually had no qualms about being called dealers. They generally had a high-school education, and were not required to have additional training. Many learned their trade through apprenticeship to an older, more experienced dealer. Until recently, there was no licensure or registration for dealers.

However, some states have recently instituted these procedures. Licensure means that the dealer has passed a written (or sometimes practical) examination. Registration means only that the dealer has paid money to the state and declared himself or herself in business as a hearing aid dealer, or, if you will, a dispenser.

For the sake of convenience, we will start using the word *dispenser/ dealer* when talking about those who used to be just plain dealers; the phrase *dispensing audiologist* will refer to an an audiologist who sells hearing aids; the term *dispenser* will be used when it doesn't make any difference.

Playing this word game won't help you make a decision on which type of dispenser to choose, however, so let's get on with the matter at hand. To whom should you go for a hearing aid? Well, if you have an audiologist's recommendation for a hearing aid, and know of a well-recommended dispenser/dealer in the area, you may get excellent service there. However, if you don't know a dispenser/dealer by reputation, you may be better off buying from a dispensing audiologist. Here's why:

- You know for sure that an audiologist has had some training in the field.
- An audiologist has been licensed by the state, accredited by a national professional group, or both.
- An audiologist will be able to do further testing later on to follow the progression, if any, of the hearing loss.
- Most dispensing audiologists will be able to handle any therapy and training you will need.
- A dispensing audiologist probably won't charge any more than a dispenser/dealer.

Again, this does not mean that a dispenser/dealer won't do a good job. There are many skilled, competent, and concerned dispenser/dealers in the marketplace; they are also easier to locate simply because there are more of them than dispensing audiologists. However, you have no guarantee that the dispenser/dealer you pick out of the yellow pages will be knowledgeable and conscientious.

On a related note: Physicians have been known, on occasion, to refer a patient directly to a dispenser/dealer. This is generally not a good practice. For one thing, a dispenser who is not an audiologist generally has no training in the complexities of hearing testing, and may not be able to spot or deal with special problems. The equipment used will probably not be as sophisticated as an audiologist's.

Regardless of whether you visit a dispensing audiologist or a dispenser/dealer, the process of fitting will be roughly the same. Fitting involves having an earmold made, adjustment of the aid and earmold, and an orientation program. Here's how the process usually works:

Step 1

The financial situation is often the first thing talked about. If not, it should be the first thing you ask about. The cost of hearing aids will be discussed later in this chapter, and related advice will be offered in Chapter 14.

Step 2

Once you've agreed on the price of a recommended aid, the dispenser—after seeing your medical clearance—will make an impression of your ear for a personalized earmold if you didn't have one made for the hearing aid evaluation. A puttylike material will be left in your ear for about ten minutes until it dries and hardens. This impression will be used to make the earmold. However, this is not a foolproof process, and the mold may not fit perfectly the first time. If you are getting an in-the-ear or canal style the hearing aid will be built into a case made from this impression.

Step 3

You should return to the dispenser in ten days to two weeks; during this time the earmold will have been ordered from a laboratory. You will now try on the earmold and the aid, or the in-the-ear aid. If any immediate adjustments are needed they will be made at this point.

Step 4

Additional hearing tests may or may not be carried out after you try on the aid and earmold for the first time. These tests typically measure how well you understand speech. Some dispensers prefer to let you become more accustomed to the aid before these tests; some dispensers don't bother at all.

Step 5

The dispenser should now give you an orientation to the aid, and work with you until you understand how to put it on and take it off, check the battery (by intentionally making the aid feed back), operate the controls, and care for the instrument. The orientation should also include hints on how to get used to the aid (such as the suggestions outlined in Chapter 6), and a recommended schedule for breaking it in. You will also at this time be given a *user instructional brochure*, which explains all these things in words and pictures. The brochure will also carry a warning about irritation from the earmold: some irritation is normal at first, but if soreness or irritation persists, the earmold must be adjusted. Also, as the brochure will explain, some people are allergic to the substance in the earmold; if that's the case, you will need to buy a special kind of mold. You will also be notified that you may experience quite a bit of wax accumulation, as explained in Chapter 6. There is one more warning in this brochure: If the output of the aid exceeds a certain level, it could cause additional hearing loss. Don't let this worry you unduly, because very few hearing aids extend to this maximum output, and if you do need this type of power the audiologist will have already discussed it with you.

Step 6

You should ask any questions you have. Be sure to take advantage of your time with the dispenser, because you are paying for this service in the cost of the aid. Whatever you do, don't pretend to understand when you really don't. If you're having difficulty with the aid in the dispenser's office, things will only get worse once you're home.

Step 7

You will probably return in the near future (within three weeks, usually) to have your progress and the hearing aid checked by the dispenser. In the meantime, you should call on the telephone or make another visit if you experience difficulty. Do not hesitate to take these opportunities if you need help; it is part of what you paid for.

Your hearing aid will probably be sold to you on a thirty-day trial basis, or with a thirty-day money-back guarantee. On the trial basis, you pay a minimal fee ($20 to $50) until after the thirty-day period; if you're not satisfied you may elect to return the aid. The thirty-day money-back guarantee follows much the same procedure, except you put up the money first. Most dispensers operate on one of these two plans, and it is worth your while to do business with one who does. Be aware that if you return the aid the dispenser will keep from $30 to $50; this amount is kept to cover cost of the earmold and the complete reconditioning the aid must undergo before it can be sold.

Now comes the big question: How much will a hearing aid cost? It varies from about $325 to $550. Most, but not all, of this variation stems from the profit margin of the dispenser, not from the wholesale price of the aid. One dispenser may charge $200 more than a competitor for the exact same hearing aid.

Part of the reason for the wide variance in price is, of course, the profit the dispenser wants to make on the deal. The other factor concerns the services offered, which are included in the total cost. When you sit down to discuss financial matters with the dispenser, it is vital that you determine what services are included. If some essential services are not part of the total price, you may not be getting the bargain you expected when you were quoted the low price. The total price should include:

- the cost of the hearing aid(s) itself
- the cost of the earmold(s)
- one pack of batteries
- any adjustments to the aid or mold
- counseling and orientation
- return visits—there will probably be at least one or two
- the warranty on the aid(s), usually for one year

These are the basic services that should be included; others may also be provided. If some extra services come with the package, you might take them into account when comparison shopping.

True, these services do drive up the cost of a hearing aid. Remember, though, that for anyone in business, time is money—and quite a bit of the dispenser's time will be spent on your testing, orientation, and return visits.

This is not to say that you shouldn't expect a good buy, especially now that you're aware of the services that should be included with the purchase price. You may wish to keep this book with you when you talk with dispensers; if they provide all the services listed, you can now compare on the basis of price alone and judge the best bargain.

If you visit or telephone several dealers, you will note from signs in the window or ads in the yellow pages that they often specialize in two, three, or four brands. If the audiologist has recommended a certain brand, you will get the best buy if you deal with a dispenser who specializes in that particular brand. When dispensers do a great amount of business with one manufacturer, they can generally get a better wholesale price. They will also be more familiar with the individual aid, and may be able to handle minor repairs themselves, without having to send the aid to the factory for service.

In any event, you will probably get the most for your money if you stick to major brands; a list of them follows. If an audiologist recommends a brand that is not on this list, it does not mean there's something wrong with the brand, or that someone's trying to pull a fast one on you. The hearing aid industry is changing rapidly, and what may be a minor brand when this list was compiled could corner the market in a few years. Just because a firm isn't a major seller, it doesn't indicate that its product is shoddy; it does mean that professionals in the field have had less experience with the product and won't place as much confidence in it as a well-known name brand.

Major Hearing Aid Manufacturers

(in alphabetical order)

Acousticon	Dahlberg	Oticon	Rion
Argosy	Danavox	Panasonic	Siemens
Audiotone	Electone	Philips	Starkey
Audiovox	Fidelity	Phonic Ear	Telex
Beltone	HSI	Qualitone	Unitron
Bernafon	Maico	RadioEar	Widex
Bosch	Omni	Rexton	Zenetron

Finally, there is one important point that must be stressed: *If you buy two hearing aids, you should not pay double the price*. Never! Remember that the price you pay includes a hefty markup for the dispenser's time. The amount of time spent in giving you an orientation and teaching you to use the aid does not suddenly double when you wear two of them. Two aids should cost in the neighborhood of $550 to $800.

Unfortunately, dispensers have been known to get away with simply doubling the price on a customer who buys two aids. To make sure you're getting a fair price, when you buy one aid or two, it's a good idea to ask the dispenser to "unbundle" the price—that is, to give you a breakdown of what each piece of the package is costing you. That way, you know exactly what you're paying for. To give you an idea of how much the dealer's markup is, bear in mind that most (not all) hearing aids wholesale to the dispenser for about $150 to $175. Dispensers are certainly entitled to a fair profit—they couldn't stay in business otherwise—but by the same token, you have a right to get your money's worth when you make such a substantial investment.

After you have purchased a hearing aid, you may want to buy one or more handy devices that make coping with your hearing loss a bit easier; some of those devices will be featured in the next chapter. First, here are some questions frequently asked about buying a hearing aid:

How do I check the qualifications of the dispenser/dealer? In a state where there is no licensure, you will have few qualifications to check on. If there is dispenser/dealer licensure in your state (ask an audiologist) the license should be posted at the dealer's office. Otherwise, you must rely upon the recommendation of an audiologist, a doctor, or perhaps a friend who has dealt with a particular dispenser.

Will one style of hearing aid, an in-the-ear, for example, cost more than other styles? The instruments themselves, except the canal aid, all cost about the same, but you will probably wind up paying more for an eyeglass aid because of the optics and the greater number of adjustments you will need for the device.

I'm going to buy a new aid soon. Will the dispenser give me a trade-in on my old aid? Very rarely. The aid won't do the dispenser any good, other than being used as a loaner after it is reconditioned; in most states, it can't be sold. You would be wise to keep the old aid as a spare. If you don't want or need it, some fraternal organizations, such as the Lions Club, will recondition the aid and give it to someone in need. Whatever you do, *don't* give the aid to a friend who has a hearing problem. Although they are not as specific as eyeglasses, hearing aids are prescribed to fit particular hearing problems. An inappropriate aid is worse than useless: It can cause so much frustration that your friend may throw it away and decide never to wear a hearing aid again.

Are all the warranties on hearing aids for only one year? A few companies now have warranties for two or even three years; however most are still for one year. For a small additional charge, some companies will extend the warranty on their aids. You can also get insurance from an independent insurance carrier for such things as loss, theft, or accidental damage. This is often not a bad idea because the warranty usually does not cover them.

[10]
Other Helpful Devices

As we mentioned before, a hearing aid is just what the name implies—an aid. It does not restore normal hearing, and there are some situations in which it may be of limited help (for example, several people all talking at once; a lot of background noise; a sermon, play, or concert; watching television; talking on the telephone). There are also times when you aren't wearing your hearing aid(s) but you still need to hear, such as when you're in bed or in the shower, and the telephone, doorbell, or smoke alarm rings, or an intruder appears. Or, you may have a loss so severe that even a hearing aid does not help you hear the sounds you want or need to hear.

This chapter is about devices beyond hearing aids that can be very helpful in the above situations. These devices can mean the difference between just getting along and a much easier and finer quality of life. They are relatively inexpensive considering the convenience and enjoyment they will afford. You deserve them.

One benefit of the American free enterprise system is the fact that there will never be a shortage of gadgets to buy. For the hearing impaired, there is a wide variety of gizmos that flash, vibrate, print, and amplify.

Most of the devices discussed in this chapter are designed primarily for people with severe hearing losses. Use of some, though, can make life a bit easier even if you might be able to get along without them. A good example of a device to make life a little easier and more enjoyable is *closed-captioned television*.

Even if you hear well enough to understand most of what's being said on your favorite shows, listening to the audio is still likely to be a strain. And trying to follow a TV show will be almost impossible if you hear very poorly. Closed captioning relieves this strain by printing out subtitles—the general idea of what's being said, as shown in Figure 8.

The NBC, ABC, and PBS television networks, as well as some independent stations, cable TV systems, and Canadian broadcasters, have been using a format called Line 21, which is used to program a collective

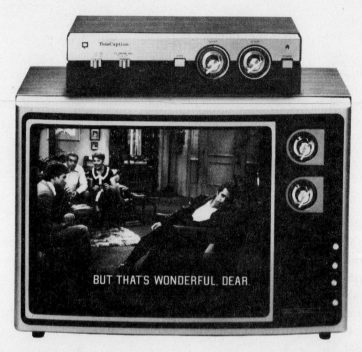

BUT THAT'S WONDERFUL, DEAR.

Figure 8. Closed-captioned television. An adaptor, placed on top of the TV, allows the viewer to read captions provided on certain programs. (Photo courtesy of National Captioning Institute, Inc.)

total of about seventy hours of closed-captioned television; you can find out which programs are captioned from most television program listings, including *TV Guide*. CBS has recently begun captioning with a different format—the North American Broadcast Teletext Standard (NABTS), where there is currently limited on-demand information (about fifty pages) such as news, weather, travel, sports, and feature services. According to the National Captioning Institute, NBC will also use NABTS primarily for the information aspect rather than the captioning aspect. The amount of closed captioning of programs for the NABTS format is minimal at the time of this writing, so dual-mode captioning was initiated by NBC and CBS; in dual-mode captioning, programs are captioned in both NABTS and Line 21.

Captions only appear if you have an adaptor. The adaptor can be turned on and off so the television can be seen without captions. The Line 21 adaptor works on any television, while the NABTS adaptor works only on specific brands (such as Panasonic, Quasar, and Pioneer).

The captions are about a half-inch high when they're on a nineteen-inch television screen. To insure legibility, the area immediately behind the captions is blacked out.

Line 21 captioning adaptors can be purchased from:

1. The National Captioning Institute, 5203 Leesburg Pike, Falls Church, VA 22041. (Western Division address: Hollywood-Gower Studios, 1438 North Gower St., Hollywood, CA 90020)
2. Sears, Roebuck and Co. and J. C. Penney Co.
3. Various organizations for the deaf.

Also, closed-caption devices can be leased through some cable system operators. There is now a cable converter/decoder for some cable subscribers. NABTS sets and adaptors are available from dealers in the particular brands of TVs for which they are available.

A Line 21 closed-caption system that can be added to your television set costs about $300. Sets with the captioning device included cost about $500 to $600.

As we mentioned, only a certain amount of television programming is closed captioned. But while not all programs are closed captioned, a wide *variety* of programs are. You will be able to enjoy closed-captioned movies, network news, situation comedies, sporting events, dramas, miniseries, children's shows, and occasional specials.

There are also home videocassette movies (Line 21 format only) that are closed captioned, such as those produced by RCA/Columbia Home Entertainment.

Remember, closed-captioning units, like hearing aids and many of the other devices useful to the hearing impaired, are tax deductible.

There are some other devices available to those who have trouble understanding the dialog on TV programs (a very common problem among people who have only mild losses, by the way; remember that the sound coming from a television speaker is distorted to begin with, and not accompanied by as many visual cues as in real life). One such device sends the audio signal directly into an earpiece worn by the hearing-impaired person. Unlike the standard earphone on a television, some of these instruments don't cut out the speaker, so others can watch television with you. The volume control for your earpiece can be adjusted separately from the TV volume control. Prices for this unit—and most of the equipment described in this chapter—vary widely, so it's a good idea to call several hearing aid dispensers (who would most likely order this type of gear from a manufacturer).

Another device for the television is a microphone hooked to an infra-red light emitter. A receiver worn by the listener picks up the light, which actually carries a sound signal from the television. The signal is amplified and played back through headphones. Now, you can hear the television well while the volume is turned to a level comfortable for others in the room. Also, remember that while you are listening under those headphones, the noise in the room around you is blocked out and won't interfere as much. An infra-red emitter and receiver can be found for as low as $300.

Many public places such as churches, theaters, and schools have installed infra-red systems for their hearing-impaired patrons. The speaker's voice or music is transmitted via infra-red light to special receivers provided by the facility. The impaired person wears the receiver and turns the volume up to a comfortable level.

Another slightly more elaborate system that is commonly used in classrooms for better reception of the teacher's voice is a radio-frequency FM system. The speaker wears a lavaliere (necklace) mike, which is also a tiny radio transmitter. The voice is carried over the air within a fifty-foot radius and is picked up by a receiver about the size of a cigarette package worn by the impaired listener. The voice is amplified and put directly into the person's ear or is routed through their hearing aid(s). The advantage is a clear, amplified sound with little background noise interference. The cost for this system for one person (mike, receiver, and recharger) is about $1,200, with about $400 for each additional receiver. This system can be invaluable to someone who must frequently listen in situations where a speaker is addressing a large group. It is transportable from place to place and easy to use.

Other helpful devices for someone with a hearing loss interact directly with the telephone. Many hearing aids are equipped with a T-switch. When the switch is in the T (for telephone) position, the aid is no longer sensitive to sound waves. Instead, it amplifies electromagnetic waves, such as the ones produced in the receiver of a telephone. The theory, of course, is that the telephone signal can be transmitted directly into the hearing aid without amplifying any background noise in the room. In practice, though, two basic problems arise:

1. When a wiretapping scare swept through the country several years ago, telephone companies installed special shields in receivers to keep a bug from picking up the signal. Unfortunately, the shielding also prevents a T-switch–equipped hearing aid from operating properly. Telephone companies are supposed to provide you with an unshielded telephone upon request. Most pay phones can be used with a T-switch. Recently, federal legislation required that all telephones for necessary communication (such as public phones) be compatible with the T-switch.

2. At best, the reception from a T-switch–equipped hearing aid is not great. There is usually some distortion and the quality of the T-circuit varies widely from aid to aid.

Even though the T-switch might not be the answer to all your telephone problems (we'll discuss some alternatives in a moment) it can be very helpful in combination with a system called a *loop*. How does a loop system work? A microphone picks up, let's say, a sermon. It then feeds the sermon through a powerful system of wires encircling the room. By switching the hearing aid to the T-position, you receive a direct feed of the electromagnetic signal, with no background noise. The reception should be better than what you get from the telephone, since the system is built specifically for this type of transmission, while the telephone is not. The loop system idea can be applied to a radio or television set, and will feed the audio into a loop around the person, and thus to the hearing aid via the T-switch.

Many churches, lecture rooms, theaters, and concert halls have installed these loop systems (or infra-red systems, such as those discussed earlier in this chapter). Most of these locations advertise this service; just ask in which section of the room you should sit. If you don't have a hearing aid with a T-switch, most places will have a receiver you can borrow, and you will be given instructions on how to use it.

But, as we mentioned, even though the T-swich on a hearing aid opens up interesting possibilities, it doesn't completely solve the problem it was originally designed for: communicating over the telephone. To be frank, most hearing-impaired people and telephones just don't get along. Use of the telephone is one of the most irksome problems faced by the hearing impaired, for a number of reasons. The biggest problem usually rests in the fact that the normal telephone just isn't loud enough.

A device to overcome this dilemma is an amplified telephone equipped with a volume wheel or switch available from the phone company. The wheel or switch, located in the center of the hand-held portion of the phone, works just like the volume control on a radio. The advantage of having a volume wheel is that you can turn the phone up as loud as you like, while getting a relatively undistorted signal.

You will, however, want to take your hearing aid off when talking into this type of phone or any phone not equipped with a T-switch (unless you can use the unaided ear). The only time it's feasible to use a hearing aid to amplify the sound of the telephone is with an in-the-ear or canal aid that is far enough inside the ear so that a tight seal can be made between the telephone earpiece and the outer ear, and even then your hearing aid may squeal.

Having to take off the aid when using the telephone is one disadvantage of the amplified telephone. There is also a charge for the installation of a volume-wheel-controlled phone (usually about $25), and a minimal per-month rental fee. Also, remember that if you depend on an amplified telephone, you are generally restricted to your own phone; however, when you see a pay phone marked for handicapped users it will generally be equipped with a volume wheel.

For about $25 you can purchase a small coupler that fits over the listening end of your telephone receiver and makes the sound louder. It is easily moved from one phone to another. However, the quality is not quite as good as a built-in amplifier, and if you forget to turn the coupler off when you hang up, the batteries wear out quickly. The couplers are often available in electronic shops.

For those who can't use a telephone at all, there's a device called a TDD, or telecommunications device for the deaf (shown in Figure 9), which transmits typewritten messages over the telephone wires.

The basic stripped-down model costs less than $300. You type your message in on a typewriter-type keyboard, and it is typed out on a screen on the receiver's TDD. You can also buy a system that prints out the conversation on paper as well. You are, of course, limited to calling parties who have a TDD, but that number may not be as small as you think. Many businesses and organizations are installing TDDs, including airlines, hospitals, fire and police stations, schools, and government offices. There are also services whereby an operator will receive the TDD message and retransmit it orally to a party who has only a conventional telephone. The

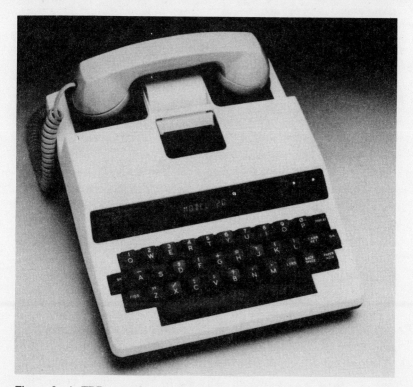

Figure 9. A TDD, or telecommunications device for the deaf. The message transmitted shows up on the screen above the keyboard. (Photo courtesy of Krown Research, Inc.)

telephone companies usually offer reduced long-distance rates when a TDD is used (because it takes longer to type than to talk). Some states have introduced legislation requiring that hearing-impaired people be able to purchase TDDs at a reduced price; you might check with your audiologist, TDD dealer, or state representative.

If your hearing loss is severe enough to require a TDD, you may also be in the market for one or more sound-sensitive visual alarms. These alarms can be made sensitive to almost any sound that you need to know about, such as a doorbell, telephone ring, an intruder, or even a human voice, such as a baby's cry. The visual alarm generally consists of a flashing light. The more complex alarm systems use your home electrical circuits to carry signals so that, without obtrusive wiring, you can have a lamp that flashes in each room. There can be a code of flashes for the different sounds around the house. For example, a telephone ring could be two short flashes; the doorbell could be three long flashes; while the stove timer might be two long and a short. Incidentally, unless you are totally deaf the best system for alerting you to an intruder would be a very loud burglar-alarm system. You can even get one that would also ring into your neighbor's house or (in many locations) to the police station, or the central station of the burglar-alarm company.

Vibrators are helpful for people who have trouble waking to an alarm clock. The vibrator usually is connected to the clock and placed under the pillow; the vibrator replaces the normal alarm buzzer on the clock. You can even have your doorbell hooked into this vibrating-clock system. But before you invest in a sophisticated wakeup system, check out some of the old-fashioned wind-up alarm clocks, such as the Baby Ben. These clocks generate quite a bit of noise and will certainly be louder than a buzzer on most electric clocks or clock radios.

There's another device that merits a mention in this chapter, although it is for people with tinnitus, which is not, strictly speaking, a hearing loss. Tinnitus, as described earlier, is a ringing or roaring sensation in the ears, and it often accompanies an age-related hearing loss, although it's not necessary to have a hearing loss in order to have tinnitus.

No one is really sure what causes tinnitus, but we do know that it's a big problem: About thirty-six million people in the United States are affected by it at one time or another. There are varying degrees of tinnitus: For some, it is a mild annoyance; for others, a very serious handicap.

Very few cases of tinnitus are medically treatable, but a device called a *tinnitus masker* can help people to live with it. The masker, which looks like a hearing aid (or may be manufactured within a hearing aid) produces a sound that is similar to the continuous rushing of water. Many tinnitus sufferers find that this external sound, while distracting, covers up the internal sensation in their ears and is far less of an irritation. For a few people, wearing the masker for a period of time will bring about a temporary end to the tinnitus even after the device is removed.

Unfortunately, after a period of time the masker may become less and less effective. Also, some people are truly annoyed by the sound over a long time. Currently under research is a device for eliminating tinnitus using electrostimulation; the person wears a headset with two electrodes for four to five hours a day. There is no sensation of sound nor is there any other sensation from the electrical stimulation. For *some people* the tinnitus stops during the procedure and for some time after.

In any event, if you have tinnitus, it's wise to check with an ENT physician first to see if there is any medical cause for it. The ENT is also the first person you'll need to contact in order to get a masker (he must give clearance, just as with a normal hearing aid).

The best way to purchase any of the assistive devices mentioned in this chapter is through a hearing aid dispenser who can tell you if your type of hearing loss is appropriate for a specific device; the dispenser may even suggest an alternative device. It is also a good idea to have a local person to whom you can turn for advice on how to set up the device, how to use it, and how to get it repaired.

Most of the devices are not sold in typical stores, except for ones like a regular burglar alarm or a coupler for your telephone.

If you do not have a local dispenser you can write or call for free information from these sources:

Better Hearing Institute
1430 K. St., N.W., Suite 600
Washington, DC 20005
Telephone: Hearing Helpline (toll free), 1-800-424-8576

NAHSA
National Association for Hearing and Speech Action
10801 Rockville Pike
Rockville, MD 20852
Telephone: Helpline (toll free), 1-800-638-8255

National Hearing Aid Society
20361 Middlebelt
Livonia, MI 48152
Telephone: Hearing Aid Helpline (toll free), 1-800-521-5247

These sources, by the way, can be very helpful to you in other ways besides giving you information on assistive devices. The Better Hearing Institute, for example, is dedicated to encouraging those with uncorrected hearing losses to get help, and to encouraging others to protect their hearing from loss. Its Hearing Helpline provides referrals to local professionals and handles questions and complaints about hearing help, hearing aids, and hearing aid services.

NAHSA is the consumer affiliate of the American Speech-Language-Hearing Association, which provides referrals and information on all aspects of communication disorders, including specific hearing problems and treatments, legal rights, and financial matters. The Consumers Organization for the Hearing Impaired is a national group committed to furthering the interests of persons with hearing impairment. It has recently affiliated with NAHSA, but retains its independent status. Its published materials can be requested on NAHSA's toll-free line, listed above.

The National Hearing Aid Society provides an information package to those who suspect they have a hearing loss, telling them what steps they should take, and supplies them with the names of certified hearing aid specialists in their area.

One final note: When you make plans to purchase any type of device, such as a hearing aid or any instrument described in this chapter, always keep firmly in mind that no gadget will be the cure-all for a hearing impairment. It may make your life easier, but it won't solve the basic communication problems that result from a hearing loss. *If you don't expect it to, you won't be disappointed.*

There are many aspects of communication that won't ever be the same, regardless of what you buy or how much money you spend. Conversation in a noisy restaurant will never be particularly easy, and it probably will always be a bit difficult to hear a distant speaker. But this doesn't mean there's nothing you can do to improve matters—far from it. By practicing a program for better communication, outlined in the next chapter, you can polish your communication skills and effectively cope with all types of everyday situations.

First, let's examine some typical questions about the topic covered in this chapter:

I read somewhere about "hearing ear dogs." Was it a joke?" Not at all. Several firms are training hearing ear dogs, usually for people who are totally deaf or have a very severe hearing loss, and live alone. The hearing ear dog is trained to be sensitive to certain noises (such as a doorbell ringing or a baby crying) and to run back and forth between the source of the noise and the dog's master.

I have trouble hearing the telephone when I'm in another part of the house. What should I do? The telephone company can install extra ringing devices in other parts of the house; or, of course, you can have another phone installed. Before you call the phone company, though, be sure that the ringing device on your present phone is turned up full blast. The adjustment is underneath the telephone, or on the back of a wall model.

The telephone company also can install a louder ringing device in your phone, or you can even get a ring at a lower pitch, which is easier for you to hear. If your loss is really bad, you may need a system where a light flashes when a telephone rings.

My husband gets angry when he talks to me from downstairs and I don't hear. Will a hearing aid help? Probably not entirely. Speech from another room is not only soft, but it is distorted. Hearing aids do not allow you to hear very soft sounds. And the distortion won't allow you to understand. Why not install an intercom system in the house so you can always be in touch?

I have tinnitus, and a masker doesn't seem to help. My doctor says there's nothing that can be done medically. Is there anything else I can try? Yes. Biofeedback and relaxation techniques have been helpful to some tinnitus sufferers. Biofeedback simply is a way to monitor the body's stress reactions and learn to control them. Since tinnitus is aggravated by stress, this system may help. Ask your physician for more information. Also, use of a regular hearing aid sometimes covers up tinnitus, and should be considered before opting for a masker.

[11]
A Program for Better Communication

The term *redundant* came into popular usage during the development of the space program; spacecraft carried two or three redundant, or backup, systems. The reason, of course, was that an astronaut circling the moon couldn't very well send to the hardware store for a spare part; extras had to be built into the system.

Nature had the same idea in mind when she designed our method of communication. Every message we receive is redundant in the sense that it is presented simultaneously in several different ways: We get some messages through hearing, others through sight, and some make sense to us because of our past experience with language and life.

Here's an example of how hearing, sight, and life experience interact to present a message in several different ways—all at the same time:

A small boy is playing with a plug in an electrical wall outlet. His mother rushes in and sharply yells "no!" The child gets the message, but in more ways than you might suspect.

1. The child *hears* the word "no," and even if he doesn't, at first, remember what it means, he senses that his mother is unhappy because of her tone of voice.
2. The child *sees* that his mother is rushing toward him. Her arms are outstretched, and she generally looks quite excited and unhappy. He also sees her rounded lips, which give a clue to the fact that she's just spoken the word "no."
3. The child knows from past *life experience*—even what little he's had—that something unpleasant usually happens when his mother looks and sounds like this. He may also have a pretty good idea by now of what the word "no" means.

What does this have to do with coping with a hearing loss? Well, it shows how many different clues are available to help us figure out communication. People with normal hearing, however, usually use only a few of these clues, and must be taught to utilize the rest. The most important aspect of a program for better communication is the realization that *you do not need to hear each and every individual sound or word to understand speech*. You can use your remaining hearing, your eyesight, and your life experience (including knowledge of the language) to communicate more effectively.

The first part of this chapter will spell out methods to use hearing, seeing, and life experience to full advantage. The culmination of smoothly blending these talents is called speechreading—the ability to use hearing, sight, and mental processes to figure out what is being said without complete information. Exercises in speechreading will be presented later in the chapter. First, let's concentrate on some hints to improve the three major methods of communication.

Hearing

As discussed before, listening is an active (rather than passive) activity for someone with a hearing loss. Someone with normal hearing actually has to make an effort to tune out unwanted noise; you, on the other hand, must make an effort to tune *in* to things you want to hear.

The most effective strategy for improving hearing skills involves avoiding or modifying situations that will make listening difficult. The most troubling of these situations is background noise. There are two reasons for this. First of all, an impaired hearing mechanism is excessively bothered by background noise. Secondly, the people around you aren't necessarily aware of this. People with normal hearing will usually understand that you will have trouble hearing if they speak in an excessively quiet voice. But these same people may take you to a noisy restaurant and have no idea why you are having trouble understanding the conversation. What seems like a quiet babble to them is—to you—a terribly distracting commotion.

The easiest way to deal with background noise is to change the situation or choose your location carefully. In a restaurant, ask for a table away from the band, the kitchen, or any other noisy spot. At home, do the obvious (but often overlooked) thing: Turn off the television or radio when you have a guest. This will make listening to conversation much easier.

Another hint for easier listening during background noise is to plan what you want to listen to. It's a natural tendency to want to hear everything that's going on, but someone with a hearing loss must make an effort to follow just *one* conversation. Before you enter a difficult listening situation, make a conscious effort to decide what and who you plan to listen to. (Even a person with excellent hearing can't actually listen to two conversations at once, and will switch back and forth between the two conversations to pick up the gist of what's being said. But this will be practically impossible for someone with a hearing loss.) Make up your mind and say to yourself: "While I'm here I will listen only to Tom, and not to the conversation going on over in the corner."

Background noise is not the only factor that creates a difficult listening situation. You must also consider the distance and direction of sound. One simple way to make things easier at home is to rearrange your furniture so that guests are nearby and facing directly toward you. This will allow better use of your vision, too.

Seeing

As mentioned earlier, everyone lipreads to a small extent when listening conditions are difficult. Mouth movements are helpful in figuring out what's being said; so are facial expressions and body movements. Chances are, you've been ignoring most of these valuable clues for many years.

However, you frequently do read lips without realizing it; check for yourself the next time you're in background noise. If you're not staring directly at the mouth of the person you're conversing with, you should be. Doing this will help you concentrate and provide visual cues to what is being said. Since we know how to produce sounds with our own mouths, we seem to have an innate ability to recognize the mouth movements of other people, even though we have no training. Training, of course, sharpens this ability: A good lipreader can recognize more than just the more obvious mouth movements.

But even a good lipreader can't pick up everything, although there's a common myth that an accomplished lipreader can follow a conversation by sight alone. This is, in almost all cases, just impossible: Seventy percent of sounds in the English language are produced within the mouth and not visible on the lips. Also, some sounds look exactly alike on the lips. An example of such *homophonous* sounds, as these are called, is *p, b,* and *m.*

Without hearing (or figuring out from context) it's impossible to tell apart the words *pat, bat,* and *mat* from lip movements.

There's another problem with lipreading: The human eye just can't work quickly enough to process speech by vision alone. The eye can only follow about eight or nine movements a second, while normal speech produces about thirteen mouth movements per second. And even if the eye could follow all these movements, there are still plenty of people who just don't move their mouths very much, or who have obscuring beards or mustaches that baffle the best lipreader. There are also the obvious problems of poor lighting and excessive distance from the speaker.

The point of all this is to show you that despite popular conceptions, lipreading is not the answer for a hearing-impaired person—not the whole answer, anyway. Lipreading can provide valuable clues, but unless you supplement lipreading with other speechreading techniques, you just won't be able to follow many conversations.

To pick up visual cues as part of the total speechreading process, it's important that you be aware of five basic groups of sounds that are visible on the lips. We speak of groups, rather than individual sounds, because of those bothersome homophonous sounds. You won't be able to differentiate among sounds in a particular group just from seeing them on the lips of a speaker, but by combining the use of other visual cues (explained a bit later) with your remaining hearing and the judgment gained through life experience, you should be able to deduce what's being said.

There are actually more than five groups of sounds, but many are extremely difficult to see, even with extensive training; however, it is extremely useful to know the five groups that can be read most easily on the lips. They are:

1. *P, b,* and *m*—made with the lips pressed together.
2. *F* and *v* are formed by bringing the upper teeth in contact with the bottom lip. Unlike the first group of sounds, the top lip does not touch the bottom lip.
3. *Th* (either the *th* in *thorn* or *therefore*) is produced with the tongue slightly protruding or immediately behind the top teeth; the lips are parted.
4. *W* and *r* are not exactly alike, but in continuous speech they are difficult to tell apart. They are formed with a rounding of the lips, and with the *w* there is a slight protrusion of the lips.

5. *Sh* and *ch* are produced with a rounding and definite protrusion of the lips, with the lips opening more than for *w* and *r*.

The best way to start learning how to lipread is to watch yourself speak in a mirror. Try to identify the sounds from the five groups (which you must memorize, so that recognition of the groups and the possible sounds within the groups becomes automatic; when you reach this stage, you will be able to keep your mind on other cues).

While you're practicing in the mirror, notice how many sounds can't be seen on the lips; *k* and *g*, for example, are formed inside the mouth. The mouth and lip position for most vowels (a, e, i, o, u) is so affected by the consonants around them that recognition is difficult. Fortunately, vowels are easier to hear because they are usually spoken somewhat more loudly. After picking up a passing acquaintance with the groups, practice with a partner using normal conversation (and the exercises in this chapter). Remember, when you're practicing conversational lipreading, have your partner use phrases or at least whole words; if just sounds are mouthed, they will look different from the way they look in normal speech.

Other than learning to identify the basic groups, the only real trick to lipreading is practice and a constant awareness of visual cues. Don't forget to observe visual cues apart from speech, by the way. A shrug, for instance, can be a helpful clue to understanding "I don't know when he will be home." A hand motion can help make sense of the statement "I left my briefcase back at the office." You will notice more and more about such mannerisms as you become aware of how they can help you understand. Indeed, you will probably be quite surprised at the amount of visual cues you overlooked when your hearing was normal.

Life Experience

Your experience, which adds up to knowledge of the language and various situations in general, is probably the most important tool you have in the speechreading process. Using life experience is essential because you're rarely going to be one-hundred-percent sure of what people are saying just by listening and looking. It is much easier to deduce what is being said if you have a knowledge of *what is likely to be said*. For example, it will be much easier to understand "pick up a pound of ground beef" if you are discussing grocery shopping. If, perhaps, you couldn't understand the beginning sound of the word *pound*, it will be obvious from the content that the word is not *mound* or *bound*.

Researchers call this process—the mind filling in the blanks—*closure*. When the mind fills in the word or sound that makes sense (a pound of ground beef rather than a mound or a bound), it's called *conceptual closure*. Another way the mind fills in incomplete information is through *grammatical closure*. If we hear a sentence that sounds like "the boy are going to the park" we can fill in the missing *s* at the end of *boy*; even though we didn't hear it we know it must be there because of the word *are* in the sentence. If it was only one boy the sentence would be "the boy *is* going to the park." This is a particularly good example, because the final *s* on *boys* is a very difficult sound for someone with an age-related hearing loss to pick up.

The point of all this is that you don't need to catch every word to understand what's being said. Your knowledge of the language and life, coupled with effective use of your remaining hearing and eyesight, can restore much of the message missed by the ears alone. However, the biggest problem faced by most hearing-impaired listeners is that they don't let the mind make effective closure; they get so hung up on trying to figure out two or three words that they forget the overall meaning of the conversation.

On the topic of overall meaning, it's important to remember that when people talk, they generally make sense. This means that if you are a secretary and your boss says what sounds like "start a new giraffe on this page," you shouldn't waste time spinning mental wheels trying to figure out why the devil a giraffe is wanted, and a new one at that. Instead, try to make an educated guess as to what could have been said that sounds like giraffe. Carafe? No, nothing's been said about wine, so that doesn't make sense. Paragraph? That's more like it.

Along the same lines, you will have an easier time making sense of conversation if, as stated before, you know what to expect. Since a great deal of everyday chitchat concerns current events, a subscription to a newspaper or weekly news magazine will be helpful, especially when the conversation turns to foreign affairs that involve unfamiliar places and names.

You will generally find that any type of conversation is easier if you prepare in advance for it, even if you only have a few seconds to do so. If the topic suddenly turns to cooking, mull over some of the words you are likely to hear (recipe, ounces); if you are asking directions from a traffic cop, think in advance of difficult words you are likely to encounter (such as intersection, expressway). Then make a special effort to recognize these words in conversation.

Try some role playing with a partner. Invent situations, such as a post office, doctor's office, or voter registration office, and have your partner make up some words that would apply to each situation. Your partner should mouth the words silently, using no voice, while you try to lipread. Notice how much easier it is to figure out *air mail* and *certified* when you know that the topic is the post office. Now that you see the value of knowing the topic in advance, you can pick situations and come up with words you are likely to hear.

For example, in a department store:

1. aisle	5. giftwrap	8. refund
2. cash	6. receipt	9. escalator
3. display	7. sale	10. brand
4. hardware		

Exercises like this are extremely valuable in enhancing speechreading skills. Here are some exercises that are commonly used in hearing therapy groups. Try and make up some of your own after you finish these.

Exercise 1: Being aware of facial expressions and gestures. Try these activities to practice getting as much information as possible from facial expressions and gestures:

- Look at photographs in magazines and newspapers and guess at what might have been said by the subject of the photo. Does the subject look angry, questioning, sad? Does the subject appear to be talking or listening?
- Watch television with the sound off. Try to imagine—from the gestures and expressions you see—what is going on and what is being said.

Exercise 2: Picking up cues from various situations. Since speechreading is really a series of educated guesses, the more possibilities you can anticipate (things likely to be said) the better. To develop the habit of giving yourself more cues to the content of the message, stop and think for a moment before you go into a familiar situation. Try to predict the things that may be said to you. You'll have a better chance of understanding conversation when you know what to expect. Using your past experience, predict what is likely to be said in the following examples (we've given a few samples; try to make up some more of your own):

Situation	What might be said
Out to dinner	How many in the party?
	Something from the bar?
	Are you ready to order?
	We have beans, carrots, and corn.
	Please pass the salt and pepper.
	I'll get the check.
At the gas station	Fillerup?
	Back up, please.
	No-lead or super no-lead?
	Should I check under the hood?
	Your right front tire looks low.
	Sorry, we don't take credit cards.
Registering at the hotel	Do you have a reservation?
	Double or twin beds?
	Sign here, please.
	The bellman will take your bags.
	Please pay the cashier when you leave.
At the bank	Can I help you?
	Is this for savings or checking?
	Do you want tens or twenties?
	Would you sign the back of the check?
	Could I see some identification?
At the doctor's	Have you been here before?
	Which doctor is your appointment with?
	Fill these out and bring them back.

Situation	What might be said
	Have you been staying on your diet?
	Describe the pain for me.
	Your insurance will not pay for this.

Exercising 3: Recognizing the homophonous groups. Go back and review what the groups of sounds look like on the lips. Following are lists of identical-looking words within each group. Have a helper say one of the words to you silently. Be sure your partner uses normal lip movements; exaggerated lip movements will only prove distracting. You should try to determine what *group* the beginning or final sound of the word is in—the *p, b,* and *m* group; the *f* and *v* group; the *th* group; the *w* and *r* group; or the *ch* and *sh* group. *Don't try to guess the word—that's impossible, and you'll only get frustrated.* Guess the *group.* For example, if your partner silently says "boot" in an exercise dealing with the beginning sound, your response should be "the p, b, and m group." If your partner silently says "bath" in an exercise dealing with the end of words, your response should be "the th group."

The only reason we are using words is that having your partner say individual sounds would be worthless, since the lip movements would be distorted. By the way, your partner should skip around among these lists; it will be a bit obvious if all the words from the *p, b,* and *m* group are said one after the other. Your partner should tell you whether the group sound you are guessing occurs at the beginning or end of the word.

Words beginning with sounds from the *p, b,* and *m* group:

BOOT	MAT	POLE	MOLE	BONE	BORE
MADE	MAKE	BAT	BEAT	MIKE	PIKE
PAT	BAKE	MORE	MUD	BUD	MEAT
PAID	POUR	BIKE	POOL	PEST	BACK

Words ending with sounds from the *p, b,* and *m* group:

LAMB	SLAB	TOM	TOP	LAP	LAB
SLIM	COP	SLAP	CALM	SLIP	SLAM

Words beginning with sounds from the f and v group:

FAN	FEND	VAULT	FAT	VENT	VAN
VEST	VINE	VAT	FINE	FAULT	FILL

Words ending with sounds from the f and v group:

LEAF	STRIFE	STRIVE	LIVE
LEAVE	SAFE	LIFE	SAVE

Words beginning with sounds from the th group:

THIS   THAT   THROW   THINK

Words beginning with sounds from the w and r group:

WING	WOUND	WAIT	WEAK	WAIL	RAIL
RATE	RUN	RING	ROUND	RAKE	WON

Words beginning with sounds from the sh and ch group:

SHOW	SHOES	SHIP	SHIN
CHIP	CHIN	CHEW	CHOOSE

Words ending with sounds from the sh and ch group:

LEASH	WISH	WHICH	MUSH
WASH	WATCH	LEACH	MUCH

Exercise 4: Guessing words. Now's your chance to guess the whole word. Below are sets of three words (note that the words are not from the same homophonous group). You choose a set of three words. Your partner will mouth one of the three words; you must select the word based on the lip movements you see.

PAY, WAY, THEY

BAT, THAT, CHAT

LIME, LIVE, LIAR

RAIL, BAIL, FAIL

BOAT, VOTE, WROTE

POUND, ROUND, FOUND

MEAT, WHEAT, CHEAT

FINE, WINE, MINE
BOO, FEW, SHOE
FAULT, VAULT, MALT
THINK, WINK, MINK
CHIN, THIN, FIN

Exercise 5: Guessing groups in a sentence. Have your partner read each of these sentences silently, mouthing the words. You are to guess which *group of sounds* appears most frequently. Do not try to guess the sentence itself.

BOB BROKE THE BOY'S BIKE.
SHE CHOSE TO SHOW HER SHOES.
THEY RODE ROUND IN THE RED ROADSTER.
PUT THE PURPLE POLE ON THE PORCH.
THE VIEW FROM THE VILLAGE IS VIVID.
WILLIAM WENT TO WATERTOWN TO WEIGH HIS WAGON.
THE FLAT TIRE WAS FINALLY FIXED ON FRIDAY.
THERE ARE THREE THOUSAND THESPIANS IN THE THEATER.

Exercise 6: Practicing grammatical closure. Your brain fills in information without any conscious effort on your part. Once you've learned a language, you apply the rules of grammar even when the message is heard incorrectly. Have your partner read the following sentences aloud— without saying the parts in parentheses. The sentences have intentional errors. The errors duplicate what people with a hearing loss might *think* they hear. Note how your knowledge of grammar enables you to correct the error without even thinking about it.

THE BOY(S) ARE GOING TO THE STORE.
THE MAN BOUGHT (A) CAR.
THAT IS SALLY('S) DRESS.
WHO (IS) COMING HOME?
HE IS GO(ING) TO THE BANK.
GIVE THE BALL (TO) JACK.
I LEFT MY KEYS (IN) MY CAR.
HE GO(ES) BACK HOME EVERYDAY.

Exercise 7: Practicing conceptual closure and flexibility. Your past experience with language and with life helps you to figure out what was said by:

a. helping you judge what might have been said, even if you didn't hear the whole message correctly

b. enabling you to eliminate choices that just don't make sense

However, in order to figure out what might have been said, you must remain open to many different kinds of possibilities—as long as they make sense. In the sentences below, fill in the blank in at least four different ways. Be flexible, and consider *all* the different possibilities; remember that there are many different shades of meaning in the English language. Some possible ways the sentence can be completed are given at the end of the exercise. See if you can come up with an equally wide range of possibilities.

a. I HAVE A BLUE _____.

b. I WENT TO _____ ON MY VACATION.

c. I DRIVE A _____.

d. I LIKE _____ SANDWICHES.

e. GET SOME _____ AT THE GROCERY STORE.

f. I FEEL _____.

g. WHERE ARE YOU _____?

h. THE BIRDS WERE _____.

Possible ways to complete the sentences:

a. sweater, car, rug, book

b. Europe, Chicago, bed, camp

c. car, motorcycle, Ford, hard bargain

d. ham, huge, fresh, club

e. milk, meat, lettuce, change

f. sad, lonely, soft, carefully

g. going, driving, at, looking

h. flying, eating, beautiful, singing

Exercise 8: Practicing flexibility and homophonous groups. Now, here's a chance to combine some skills. Following are some sentences that don't make sense—but let's pretend this is the way you heard them. For each one, first decide why it doesn't make sense. Then replace one of the words in the sentence with one that would look like it on the lips (same homophonous group) but will be more sensible. The correct replacement words are shown at the end of the exercise.

  a. DID YOU TAKE A MATH?
  b. THAT MAN IS VAT.
  c. I LOST MY CHEW.
  d. I DON'T LIKE TO RATE.
  e. SHOP THE ONIONS INTO PIECES.
  f. THE TRAIN CAME OFF THE WAIL.
  g. SOMEONE CALLED A COB.
  h. SIT ON HIS LAB.
  i. WE HAD A VINE TIME.
  j. THAT WAS VERY LEAN BEAT.
  k. I'VE HAD TOO MUSH OF IT.
  l. SHE IS REALLY GETTING SLIP.
  m. THE BIRD HURT HIS RING.
  n. THE DOG SHOULD BE ON A LEECH.
  o. PUT THE SOUP IN THE POLE.

Replacement words:

a. bath	e. chop	i. fine	m. wing
b. fat	f. rail	j. meat	n. leash
c. shoe	g. cop	k. much	o. bowl
d. wait	h. lap	l. slim	

Exercise 9: Practicing association. Fortunately, most people carry on a conversation so that the same topic is maintained for a period of time. Once you know the topic, using your past experiences you can predict what ideas and words might appear later in the conversation. Again, once you expect something, it is easier to figure out. A change in topic, of course, may throw you. Possibly you can prearrange a signal with a close companion. If the companion is talking he or she can verbally alert you to a topic change,

such as "On another topic . . ." If a third person is talking, the companion can use a signal such as touching you in a certain way to indicate a topic change.

Given the following topics, think of at least ten words or ideas that might also be heard in the conversation. Don't be rigid—think of varied possibilities as shown in the lists at the end of the exercise.

   a. BASEBALL   c. GARDEN   e. ILLNESS
   b. FOOD   d. INFLATION

Words that might be heard:

a. bat, score, little league, stadium, run, hot dogs, beer, Yankees, strike, TV

b. dessert, diet, store, refrigerator, recipe, roast beef, cost, cook, splurge, cookbook

c. plant, rain, weeds, rototiller, flowers, fertilizer, seeds, rake, vegetables, bees

d. interest, banks, bills, Congress, prices, social security, economy, stock market

e. arthritis, medicine, hospital, bed, bills, doctors, pain, aspirin, fever, heart

Exercise 10: Understanding key words. Remember that because of your hearing loss and the limitations of lipreading, it is impossible to perceive every single sound or word in a conversation. But also remember that it isn't necessary to get everything to figure out the meaning of the message.

You are looking for ideas, not words. If you try to see/hear every word you will be hopelessly lost, because while you are trying to figure out some words the speaker will get ahead of you. You are not required in conversation to repeat exactly what is said; you only need to react to ideas. So concentrate on following ideas, not words. Once you have gotten a few key words, you can figure out the rest. Pick out the three or four key words in each of the following sentences. The answers are given at the end of the exercise.

a. JOHN CAUGHT THE THIEF YESTERDAY.

b. THE LITTLE BOY CRIED BECAUSE HE LOST HIS CAT.

c. THE FAST CAR HIT THE TRUCK.
d. HER CAT CHASED THE GREY SQUIRREL.
e. THE GIRL OPENED THE DOOR SLOWLY.

Key Words:
   a. John, caught, thief
   b. boy, cried, lost, cat
   c. car, hit, truck
   d. cat, chased, squirrel
   e. girl, opened, door

Exercise 11: Using key words. Now, you can practice what you must do with the key words. Let's pretend that you only heard the following key words. For each item, give at least one—or maybe two—possible sentences that could include the key words. In conversation you would know which sentence is correct based on the context. Some possible sentences are given at the end of the exercise.

a. ANN	BAKED	APPLE	PIE
b. JOHN	STORE	YESTERDAY	
c. BOOK	ON	FLOOR	
d. PUT	FLOWERS	VASE	
e. BOOKSHELF	OVER		
f. YOU	READ	PAPER	
g. WHAT	ON	TV	
h. TURN	LIGHT	OFF	
i. ANOTHER	LOG	FIRE	
j. SALLY	SWAM	LAKE	

Possible sentences:
   a. Ann baked an apple pie.
   b. John went to the store yesterday.
      John bought a coat at the store yesterday.
   c. The book fell on the floor.
      The book is on the floor.
   d. Put the flowers in the vase.
      Put some flowers in that vase.

e. The bookshelf fell over.
   The bookshelf is over there.
f. Did you read the paper?
   You read the paper every day.
g. What's on TV tonight?
   What did you put on the TV?
g. Please turn the light off.
   Did you turn the light off?
i. Put another log on the fire.
   Another log fell off the fire.
j. Sally swam across the lake.
   Sally swam in the lake.

Exercise 12: Completing related sentences. Here is a chance to practice associating words and topics. Following are pairs of sentences that might follow each other in a conversation. Complete the second sentence using the topic of the first, word association, and your past experiences. For the first item one way of completing the sentence is given as an example.

a. I WENT TO THE STORE TO GET OLIVES.
   THEY DIDN'T have any green ones.
b. WE SAW THAT MOVIE LAST WEEK.
   I THOUGHT IT _____.
c. WHO DID YOU VOTE FOR?
   I DECIDED NOT _____.
d. THE RECIPE CALLS FOR TWO TABLESPOONS OF CORNSTARCH.
   I HAD TO USE _____.
e. THE FLOWERS WERE WILTED.
   THE WEATHER _____.

Exercise 13: Forming related sentences. This time give an entire sentence that might follow the first one in conversation based on the first sentence's topic. The first item is completed as an example.

a. DID YOU READ THE PAPER THIS MORNING?
   (The president's speech was in it.)
b. TV SHOWS ARE GETTING POORER EVERY YEAR.

   c. THE CAR SQUEALED ITS TIRES ON THE CORNER.

   d. I LEFT THOSE COOKIES ON THE TABLE.

   e. THE LIBRARY BOOKS ARE THREE DAYS OVERDUE.

Exercise 14: Speechreading related sentences. Find your partner again and practice a lot of these skills together. Following are more related sentences. Your partner should read the first one aloud and then only mouth silently the second one. Using your skills of association, watching the lips, and filling in (closure), try to get the general meaning of the second sentence.

   a. THE PAPER BOY IS HERE.
       DO YOU HAVE ANY MONEY?

   b. IT'S COLD IN HERE.
       PLEASE SHUT THE WINDOW.

   c. WE'RE HAVING POTATOES FOR DINNER.
       DO YOU WANT THEM MASHED OR BOILED?

   d. IT'S A BEAUTIFUL DAY TODAY.
       I MADE A PICNIC LUNCH.

   e. MY CAR WOULDN'T START TODAY.
       THE BATTERY MUST BE WEAK.

   f. MY SOCIAL SECURITY CHECK CAME.
       I'M GOING TO THE BANK.

   g. IS THERE ANYTHING GOOD ON TV?
       I LIKE SOAP OPERAS.

   h. WOULD YOU LIKE A SNACK?
       I HAVE SOME POPCORN.

   i. I'M HAVING TUNA FISH FOR LUNCH.
       I ALWAYS EAT FISH ON FRIDAYS.

   j. I'M WORKING IN THE GARDEN.
       I LOVE TO PLANT FLOWERS.

Exercise 15: Listening practice. You need to practice listening with your new hearing aid(s). There are some sounds that will probably be very difficult for you. Following are some pairs of words that sound similar. Sit next to your partner and hold the book in front of you so you can see the words but so that you can't see your partner's face. Listen as one of each pair of words is read aloud to you. Try to determine which one was said. Practice a lot.

FEW, CHEW	SHOW, FOE
FIN, CHIN	SHORE, FOUR
FILED, CHILD	SHADE, FADE
FOUR, CHORE	LEASH, LEAF
FIT, KIT	ICE, EYES
FOUR, CORE	BUS, BUZZ
FIND, KIND	LICE, LIES
LAUGH, LACK	SEAL, ZEAL
LEASE, LEASH	FIVE, FIFE
SEW, SHOW	VASE, FACE
SIGH, SHY	LEAVE, LEAF
SAVE, SHAVE	VIEW, FEW
TAIL, PAIL	FINE, SIGN
CAT, CAP	FLAT, SLAT
CUT, CUP	CUFF, CUSS
TOLL, POLE	NICE, KNIFE
THIN, FIN	TIE, THIGH
THIRST, FIRST	TIN, THIN
THREE, FREE	MIT, MYTH
THOUGHT, FOUGHT	PAT, PATH
KICK, TICK	PIKE, PIPE
KITE, TIGHT	CAT, PAT
CODE, TOAD	CRY, PRY
PARK, PART	COAL, POLE
THUMB, SUM	THAN, VAN
PATH, PASS	THAT, VAT
THING, SING	THINE, VINE

These exercises, and ones you might invent later on, will be quite helpful in improving communication skills. However, it's also important to learn how to pinpoint the cause of a problem.

One of the most productive self-help activities for occasions when you're having trouble hearing is *to analyze exactly where the problem lies*. A breakdown in communication can't always be blamed on your hearing loss alone.

Figure 10 shows a model of how communication occurs; this will help you locate where the breakdown happens—so that you can decide on a method of helping yourself.

First, let's look at what could be wrong with the *speaker* and what to do about it. There are some people who speak very softly or very rapidly. They may also look down or away from you while speaking. Others mumble or don't speak clearly. The solution with a speaker problem is to let these people know that there is a problem. Be polite; take some of the blame on yourself.

"Excuse me," you might say, "I don't hear that well. Could you speak a little louder (more slowly, etc.)?"

Other problems involve people with a foreign accent. You can't ask them to get rid of that, but be aware that your problem in understanding isn't all your fault.

The *message* that you are listening to may be the problem. If a message is long, uninteresting, or complex, it will be much more difficult to hear and understand. There isn't much you can do here, except to choose your conversations carefully. However, it does help to know why you have trouble following one conversation and not another.

You can try to head off the problem with some messages by preparing in advance. If, for example, the message is a lecture, sermon, or similar presentation, find out the topic ahead of time and bone up on the subject.

The environment is an area where you have a great deal of potential for change. Communication breakdown can occur when you are far away from the speaker, when obstacles keep you from seeing the person's face, when the light source is behind the speaker's face and causing a shadow, when your hearing is blocked out by background noise or multiple talkers, or when there is a distorted public-address system.

In these situations, you first have to take responsibility for your own

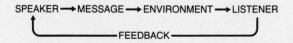

Figure 10. A communication model that can be used to analyze communication breakdown.

hearing loss by making all the changes you can. Move closer to the speaker, change your position so there are no obstacles blocking your vision, turn off the radio or television in the background, or ask for a seat away from the noise. Always arrive places early so you have a choice of seats. Once you have done all you can, politely ask others for assistance. "I am having trouble hearing you. Could you move away from that light so I can see your face? (Could you take the cigar out of your mouth? Move to the next room away from the noise? Face me when you talk? Tell me when my flight is announced?)"

Most people are quite willing to help you, but they might have to be reminded after a while. Often, by altering the environment, you can eliminate the communication breakdown, and your hearing loss won't be so much of a handicap.

Next, let's look at the problems within you, the *listener* (besides the fact that you have a hearing loss). You may have an improperly functioning hearing aid, or even none at all. You could also have poor eyesight, making lipreading difficult. What about times when you are just not interested or motivated to listen and thus have poor attention or concentration on the listening task? Perhaps you have poor skills in speechreading, or are not using your knowledge to help figure out the message.

Most of these problems can be helped by a visit to an audiologist who can fix your aid or supply one and give therapy for proper listening skills. However, it is up to you to check your eyesight, and to be aware when you are "tuning out" a conversation due to a lack of interest or motivation.

Remember that all the aspects of this chapter—speechreading, exercises to improve speechreading ability, and methods of analyzing communication breakdown—may be of more help to you if you use them in conjuction with assistance by professionals. The next chapter will explore how professionals can help you expand on self-help strategies. First let's consider some of the more frequently asked questions about these methods of improving communication.

Because I have trouble communicating, I sometimes feel as though people are walking all over me because I can't get my point across. Why do I feel this way? Maybe it's because people actually are walking all over you. The world has no shortage of insensitive boors. However, you have a right to communicate, so don't be reluctant to assert yourself. Methods of improving assertiveness will be discussed in Chapter 13. Remember, too, that some of the responsibility rests on your shoulders. You have the responsibility to learn to speechread, to get a hearing aid and learn how to use it, and to be willing to inform other people that you have a hearing problem. Once people are aware that you can't hear well, they are much more likely to make a special effort to communicate.

I'm afraid of making stupid mistakes in conversation. What can I do?
Relax. Admittedly that's easier said than done, but it's essential to learn to laugh at yourself. If, for example, you're at a restaurant, and make an odd mistake in conversation, two things can happen.

1. You can smile and say, "Sorry, I have a little trouble hearing when there's a lot of noise in the background."
2. You can fume about your mistake, and make your companion so petrified of talking to you that the conversation grinds to an immediate halt.

There's another advantage to maintaining an easy-going attitude: Your mind works much more efficiently when it's not stricken with anger or panic. You will have a better chance of understanding conversation if you are able to be flexible, and allow yourself the opportunity to think calmly.

[12]
Hearing Rehabilitation
and Therapy

After spending some time on the exercises in the previous chapter, you probably now realize the value of that type of activity in polishing speechreading skills. Whether it was apparent or not, each exercise gave you practice in doing the things necessary for good speechreading: recognizing groups of sounds in conversational speech, filling in the blanks when you don't have complete information, and learning to anticipate what sort of things might be said in some conversations.

But perhaps you really don't feel that you benefitted from the exercises, and maybe you're right. Some people just don't do well in self-help situations; they may need extra explanation, or additional motivation, or help in avoiding bad habits. Some hearing-impaired adults also don't happen to have a partner with whom they can practice.

So if you don't feel comfortable with the progress you've been making, it might be wise to investigate hearing therapy. The first step is to find a hearing therapist—an audiologist (or sometimes a speech-language pathologist) who has experience and interest in the field of aural rehabilitation. Not all audiologists and speech-language pathologists do hearing therapy, by the way. Some only do diagnostic testing, for example, or educational work with youngsters. But hearing therapists are not all that hard to find, and you can locate one by using the same guidelines used for finding an audiologist; they are outlined in Chapter 8.

If you can't decide whether or not to pursue a hearing therapy program, here are some points to consider:

- Exercises, such as the ones in the previous chapter, should be an ongoing process. In other words, you can't benefit by doing the same exercise forever. Some people have no trouble coming up with new exercises, but others just aren't that creative. A therapist, though, will have an extensive supply of exercise material.
- Working on your own may be very productive, but there's always the chance that you will get something wrong and practice a bad habit. A

151

therapist is trained to recognize a bad habit and help you alter it before it becomes ingrained.

- There are some communication skills that are impossible to present in a book and practice at home (listening practice in controlled background noise, for example). A therapist will have equipment and materials to help you practice these skills.

- A hearing therapist is trained in counseling, and can help you deal with emotional problems. The therapist will also help with problems related to your hearing aid.

- If you go to group therapy, which is cheaper and often felt to be more effective, you will meet many people who share your problem. This will often prove to be very helpful, because you can learn a lot from the experience of others.

The choice, though, is yours. You may make perfectly good progress on your own; but on the other hand, you may become stalled, and require some external motivation to keep making progress. This chapter should, at the very least, give you some idea of what hearing therapy programs are like, and what to expect from them.

What goes on in hearing therapy? Well, a typical session lasts from one to two hours, and usually takes place once a week. Sometimes, a client meets alone with the therapist, but more often the sessions involve a group of four to ten. Group sessions are most common at colleges and rehabilitation centers; these are the first places you might consider looking for a group. Hearing therapy is typically not a long-term affair, and the group will probably meet for only six to ten weeks.

The content and style of group sessions varies quite a bit, naturally. Some sessions are highly mechanical, focusing almost entirely on lip movements. If the sessions are going to deal only with lipreading, consider passing them by. They are likely to be quite boring, and of limited value. You will benefit most from sessions where a wider group of techniques (including closure, for example) are taught.

Counseling is an important part of hearing therapy, too. Although counseling can not completely take the place of training in communication skills, learning to deal with emotional problems is vitally important.

The best kind of hearing therapy involves a little of everything: practice in reading expressions, closure, lipreading, advice in dealing with emotional problems, and so forth. The goal of hearing therapy should be to mesh all these aspects.

If you do decide to join a hearing therapy group (using the above suggestions to find one that's right for you) here are some ways to insure that you get the most from your sessions:

- Make it a point to interact with the other people in your group. Learning from others is valuable. Your sessions will also become more productive after you make friends with the other participants and become more comfortable with them.
- Feel free to offer suggestions to the therapist, who is probably quite interested in how you feel the sessions could be improved. In fact, it's not uncommon for therapists to conduct a poll of their clients, seeking their reactions and suggestions.
- If you have trouble hearing the therapist, *say so*. No one will be offended. If you have a very severe hearing loss and experience a great deal of difficulty in group situations, maybe you would be better off in individual therapy.
- Planning on buying an aid in the near future? It might be best to purchase it before you start therapy. You can still attend most therapy sessions if you don't yet have an aid, but since some of the therapy will involve learning to use the aid, your time will obviously be better spent if you have one. But if you can't afford an aid right now, or have some other compelling reason why you can't get one, don't automatically pass therapy by. You can still benefit.

How much should you expect to pay for hearing therapy? Prices vary quite a bit, but in most cases, you must plan on spending at least $15 per hour for individual therapy. In group sessions the cost is often split among the members; sometimes, a flat fee is charged to each member of the group.

You'll have to decide for yourself if therapy is worth that much to you. To help you in your decision, here are three case histories. Remember that these are the best of the best examples, and not everyone can make the same kind of progress. However, these case histories do illustrate the way therapy sessions deal with emotional, social, and vocational problems.

Case History 1: An Emotional Problem

Andy was very depressed about his hearing loss, and suffered from all the typical emotional difficulties: a feeling of isolation, a suspicion that people were persecuting him, and a generally pessimistic attitude toward life. Andy's wife eventually convinced him that group hearing therapy might be a good idea. The turning point for Andy came when he realized that all the people in the session had gone through the same kind of problems. Once he knew that he wasn't alone, it was easier for Andy to make a positive effort to break the depression cycle.

Case History 2: A Social Problem

Anna's hearing loss progressed to the point where she was having difficulty understanding people in group situations. As a result of this frustration, she quit all of her clubs, and she and her husband stayed home all the time. To make matter worse, Anna let her husband take over all the communication chores, such as answering the telephone and doorbell, talking to friends, and doing household business. Eventually, she got sick of this situation and decided to join a hearing therapy group offered at the local university. After a few sessions, Anna began to realize that the answer was not *giving up* her social life, but *altering* it. Acting on suggestions from her therapist and other people in the group, Anna decided to:

- Go to quiet meetings, sit close to the front of the room, and tell the people running the meeting that she doesn't hear well and would appreciate it if they spoke up.
- Practice using her hearing aid more efficiently, to be better able to cope with social situations.
- Concentrate on lipreading exercises to help her understand more in noisy places.

Once she knew how to modify the things in life that gave her trouble, Anna found that she was once again enjoying herself. What happened recently is a good example of how she's learned to cope: A business acquaintance of her husband's wanted to get a few people together for dinner at a local restaurant. Instead of going to the noisy restaurant (it had a band) and straining all night to pick up threads of the conversation, Anna asked if it was all right to have a quiet dinner at her home, instead. No one objected, of course, and Anna had a fine time.

Case History 3: A Vocational Problem

Fay, a receptionist, was having a terrible time hearing people talk to her, especially over the telephone. Even though she was only fifty-six, Fay decided that it was time to retire. But retirement didn't turn out to be what she expected. Fay rapidly grew bored, and the loss of income really hurt. Finally, motivated more out of boredom than anything else, Fay joined a hearing therapy group she'd heard about. To her surprise, Fay found that over half the participants in the group still worked, many of them in jobs much like her own. Her therapist felt there were many jobs Fay could undertake, and referred her to the state vocational rehabilitation service. That agency helped her pay for a hearing aid (more information on vocational rehabilitation in Chapter 14) and also helped her get a job at a quieter office, where she would have the use of an amplified telephone. Fay is back at work and making money, and her newly acquired communication skills are enabling her to interact with people more frequently and effectively.

Once again, these case histories are among the most positive outcomes of thousands of cases. But good things do happen—if you make the initial effort. Whether you rely entirely on self-help material from this book or join a group, the important thing is that you recognize the need for change and take action.

The next chapter will deal with ways to take what you've learned and apply it to the real world, especially in difficult situations. First, let's examine some of the most commonly asked questions about the material in this chapter.

How can I tell if the self-help program in this book isn't working for me?
First of all, there's no reason why you can't combine the material in this book with visits to group or individual therapy, unless, of course, you live in a small town where there are no audiologists to help you. If you want to try and sharpen your communication skills on your own, give it a month or

so. If you don't feel you've made adequate improvement by then, start looking for a therapist.

You mentioned that colleges are a good place to look for a hearing therapy group. If I go to a college, won't I have a student therapist practicing on me? Sometimes, but remember that a student therapist will be closely supervised by a certified audiologist, and since the work is being done for a grade, the student is likely to make every effort to do a good job. In any event, the student's supervisor—whose business it is to train others—is likely to be a top-notch audiologist who wants to make sure you are getting useful therapy sessions.

Which is better, group or individual therapy? For most people, group therapy is probaby the better alternative, at least initially. It is less expensive and puts more emphasis on social interaction—which is what it's really all about. As mentioned before, someone with a really severe hearing loss will have a tough time in group therapy; so will someone with great emotional problems. Individual therapy is probably better for them.

[13]
Out in the World

No matter how much your communication skills improve, don't forget that even the most carefully rehearsed exercise can go astray in a real world situation. The person you're speaking with may be apathetic, uneasy, or downright hostile.

When this happens, it's time to call up what may be the most valuable trait a hearing-impaired person can develop. You must be assertive.

What is assertive behavior? Put simply, assertiveness is standing up for your own rights, but not stepping on other people in the process. This differs from passive behavior (where you let people take advantage of you) and aggressive behavior (where you violate the rights of others).

Here's why standing up for your rights is important:

- Because you have a hearing loss, you must be more assertive than most other people simply to insure that you can communicate.
- Because of your communcation problem, there will be times when others try to take advantage of you.
- You need to feel good about yourself. This won't happen if you continually are passive or aggressive.

The last point may be the most important. As we've seen, a hearing loss is tough enough on the emotions. The problem need not be compounded by a lack of self-respect brought on by passive or aggressive behavior. Two case histories help illustrate why passiveness and aggressiveness won't help your self-image.

Case History of Passive Behavior

Vera dealt with her hearing loss by nodding and smiling a lot, even though she usually didn't have the faintest idea of what was being said. Because she didn't insist on her right to communicate, Vera felt badly about herself. "I let people take advantage of me all the time," she thought. "That clerk yesterday ignored me for ten minutes, even though he knew I was waiting.

If I just didn't have so much trouble hearing, I would have spoken up."
This type of behavior led to even more passiveness, because every day
Vera would *reinforce* her self-image by her inability to cope with everyday
situations. She became trapped in a never-ending cycle.

Case History of Aggressive Behavior

Hans always got his way—regardless of how he hurt the feelings of others.
If, for example, he couldn't make out what his wife had just said, he would
snap: "Why the hell can't you speak up?" Hans found that in most cases
this type of behavior enabled him to get his way, but there was an
unfortunate side affect. People didn't like the way he acted, and avoided
him. Even his wife began to sidestep conversation as much as possible. As
a result, Hans began to feel isolated and lonely. Even though he prided
himself on always getting his way, Hans, eventually, was the loser.

Now let's see how taking the middle ground can pay off.

Case History of Assertive Behavior

Christine, a business woman, had learned that she could usually get what
she wanted by directly expressing how she feels and what she needs; in
business matters she expressed herself in an *appropriate manner*. When
she first noticed her hearing loss, Christine decided that coping with it
would require much the same approach. She not only held a high regard for
her own rights, but respected the rights of others as well. When she entered
a difficult listening situation, Christine would be likely to say: "Sorry, I
don't hear as well as I used to. Would you mind speaking up a bit?" By this
statement, Christine indicated that although she would like the other person
to speak up, she realized that the hearing loss was her problem, and she
was willing to take responsibility for it. This approach didn't always work,
by the way. Christine knew from long experience that some people will
refuse to be helpful regardless of what approach you take. But in most
cases, Christine knew that people would respect her needs if she made an
effort to respect theirs. And in any event, she would always know that she
had tried, and as a result, *she felt good about herself.*

* * *

Remember that your attitude and the way people react to you isn't based entirely on what you say; how you say it and what gestures and mannerisms you use also play a role. For example, you will frequently have to ask people to repeat things. The way in which you make the request will play an important part in determining how successful you are. Make an effort *not* to say "what? . . . what? . . . what?" It can be enormously irritating to the person you're talking with. Instead, repeat back what you've heard of the sentence so far: "John took his car and went where?" Or, "You went to the restaurant and had what?"

Not only is this approach more polite than "What? . . . what? . . . what?"; it also shows that you are interested in what is being said and it lets the speaker know how much has to be repeated. A common misunderstanding others will have about you is that you are daydreaming and not interested in following the conversation. You know that this isn't so, but it's your responsibility to make others aware of it, too. Using this method also means that the speaker won't have to repeat everything, just the part you didn't hear.

Responsibility plays a large role in coping with hearing loss. As part of assertive behavior, you must be willing to shoulder a number of responsibilities, such as:

1. *Changing or modifying your environment whenever possible.* If your living-room furniture is not arranged so that you can easily see the faces of your guests, or the light is in your eyes rather than on their faces, it is your responsibility to rearrange the furniture. It is not your guests' responsibility to go through all sorts of awkward activities so that you can see and understand them. Likewise, you are responsible for getting and learning to use a hearing aid.

2. *Changing your behavior if necessary.* Observe how you function in various situations, and work to change your behavior if it causes you difficulty. Notice how people react to you; if you want people to react differently, try to identify what it was that you said or did to cause their original reaction. If it's something that you can change and want to change, do it.

3. *Admit that you don't hear well.* Many awkward situations develop when someone refuses to admit to a hearing problem. Remember, sooner or later your hearing loss will become obvious to people

around you. If you don't admit to an obvious problem you are, in effect, telling others that you are ashamed of it. If that's the case, people around you may follow your lead and feel ashamed of it, too. But if you admit the problem in the first place, and enlist the help of others, they can give you a lot of assistance without anyone being embarrassed. Also, they won't misconstrue your behavior when they know that you have a hearing loss. They'll know that you're not a snob, that you're not stupid, and that you're not trying to hide something.

By meeting these responsibilities head on, many situations that are currently awkward for you may become easier to deal with. For example, dealing with bank tellers and store clerks can be made easier if you take the responsibility to tell them you are having trouble hearing, and then tell them what they can do to help. Someone whose job it is to communicate will usually be very receptive to suggestions on how to make things go better ("Could you speak more slowly, please, and face me?").

Although many hearing-impaired people report problems with bank tellers and store clerks, using the telephone seems to be the most vexing problem. It is your responsibility to do everything you can to modify your environment and make telephone usage easier (such as getting an amplified telephone or a T-switch on your hearing aid). But after doing your part, it's not out of line to ask others for help.

The easiest way for someone to help you understand telephone conversation is to spell out the word you are having trouble with. (Remember, problems in communication often develop because of just one or two words you can't understand. Once those words are cleared up, the conversation can move along.)

Will the person on the other end of the line think it strange that you've asked him to spell out a word? Not very likely; everyone occasionally has trouble understanding over the telephone because of the instrument's inherently poor transmission. If you walk into a police station, where critical information is constantly being taken over the phone, you'll find that everyone asks for words to be spelled out. "That's May Street, M-A-Y?" "The victim's name is spelled with a C like in Charlie, A like in Adam . . . ?"

If you have really severe difficulty using the phone, it might be wise to set up this simple, proven system with friends and family: Repeat each word. If you are talking to your son, for example, he might be able to help you understand by saying, "I-I, won't-won't, be-be, home-home, until-until, six-six." Military radio operators use this method; they ask for "words twice" when reception becomes poor.

Many hearing-impaired people have particular difficulty using the phone in an office or shop, where background noise is often very troublesome. In some cases, you may be able to ask your employer for an amplified telephone. At the very least, try to get people in your work area to recognize your need for relative quiet when taking a phone call.

Problems in the workplace won't end with the telephone. Because of the high level of background noise, it may be tough to understand conversation. There's not always much you can do about this (you can't very well ask people to stop work altogether) but if you ask co-workers for some help you will probably get it.

Following is a guide to dealing with hearing loss in the workplace. You may wish to clip these pages and keep them in your desk or locker; they contain some specific hints that we hope will be valuable. You might even wish to show this section to your employer or co-workers. First, let's list some of the most common problems encountered in the workplace. Then we'll list some possible solutions.

Common Problems in the Workplace

Background noise can be very bothersome, as mentioned earlier.

Multiple talkers are often encountered in a work area.

Talking on the telephone is difficult for most hearing-impaired people in any situation, but work can compound the problem because of noise in the environment and the need for greater accuracy in a business conversation (as opposed to a social telephone conversation).

Talking through windows (such as in a bank) or across desks makes communication difficult for people with hearing impairments.

Using earplugs or hard hats can be difficult with hearing aids. The earplug problem is obvious; a hard hat may not fit well because of a behind-the-ear aid and it may cause any aid to squeal.

Getting exact information is difficult on the phone, as mentioned, and is also a problem in face-to-face conversations. While you can afford to miss a few words in most social conversations, you must be completely accurate when taking a client's order.

Meetings pose particular difficulty because of the need to hear people all around you.

Doing things while listening is tough for people with hearing impairments. For instance, a particular task may force you to look away from the person who's speaking, and will prevent you from picking up some visual cues. It's also difficult just from the standpoint of concentration.

People not facing you causes similar problems. Often, those people will be doing things while talking.

Possible Solutions to Workplace Problems

Binaural hearing aids, as pointed out in Chapter 6, will generally improve your hearing and allow you to get more exact information. They are particularly helpful at work, where they can make multiple-speaker situations easier and help you hear from both sides in meetings.

Telephone amplifiers can help you hear better while talking on the phone and also help to tune out background noise.

A quiet office isn't always an option, but letting employers and co-workers know of your needs may result in some easily made changes that will help you function better in the office environment.

FM systems. If your work situation involves hearing one person at a time, and there is noise and distance between you, a wireless FM microphone and receiver may help greatly.

Moving away from a source of noise may be a simple solution to some of your problems. Moving your desk away from the air conditioner, for example, might be worthwhile.

Using your hearing protection will help you maintain what hearing you have. Don't believe that "more noise can't hurt"—it can.

Ask co-workers to talk one at a time. This will enable you to understand better (and might help everybody get things done more efficiently, anyway).

Use a tape recorder at meetings rather than trying to take notes. You will be able to watch the speaker's face, and you will get more complete information by playing the tape back later than you would get from notes.

Ask for preferential seating. Try to sit up front at meetings and presentations. Get there early so you have a choice.

Be assertive; you have a right to communicate.

Organize a training session for co-workers, during which you will explain how they can help you communicate. Your audiologist may be willing to conduct the training session or at least provide you with the information that should be presented. Your place of employment or the vocational rehabilitation office may be willing to pay any fee requested.

Here's an outline of what you might present during such a meeting:

Agenda: Discussion of Hearing Loss

1. The limitations of a hearing aid: It doesn't restore normal hearing.
2. The limitations of speechreading: No one can pick up all sounds from visual cues.
3. When I can and can't hear: Hearing is relatively easy in some situations, difficult in others.
4. How my co-workers can make communication easier:
    a. talking more loudly but not shouting

    b. talking at a slower pace, but not so slowly that it's unnatural

    c. facing me when they talk

    d. turning off noise sources

    e. speaking to me one at a time

    f. coming closer to me when they talk

5. Why even mild noise makes it difficult for me to hear and understand.

6. Dialog among co-workers about problems due to the hearing loss.

In some cases, these suggestions, coupled with effective hearing aids and therapy, may help you keep your present job. If you can't continue in your present position, you may have to retrain for another job.

State governments have departments that can help you keep your present job or retrain for another. These departments are usually called vocational rehabilitation agencies; check with your local social service agency to find out more.

The process for getting help from a vocational rehabilitation agency begins with filing an application. The agency will do an evaluation of your skills and attitudes. The agency may then provide counseling, prosthetic devices (such as hearing aids), and therapy.

If officials of the vocational rehabilitation agency decide that you can not continue in your current job, they will provide training for a new job, and help in job placement. They may follow up after you have been placed in a new job, to help during the adjustment period.

We hope the above suggestions help you to cope with the particular problems encountered in the workplace. One suggestion bears particular relevance to both social and vocational situations, so it might be worth repeating. Keep a pencil handy, along with a small pad of paper or a pocket notebook. When you get into the inevitable situation where there's a lot of background noise—and you just can't make out those one or two key words—take out your paper and pencil and ask the person with whom you are speaking to write those words down. Embarrassing? Maybe a little, at first. But ask yourself which will be more embarrassing in the long run: asking people to jot down the words you can't understand, or asking them to repeat the statement three or four times until you get the message—if you ever do? The pad and paper approach is definitely a convenience, and you can keep pads and pencils all through the house and workplace, as well as in your pocket.

The next chapter will deal with another aspect of real-world problems—money. But before moving on, here are some of the most frequently asked questions about dealing with difficult people and situations:

The other day I told someone about my hearing loss and he got so embarrassed he could hardly talk. Will this happen all the time? No. This reaction is rare, but it does happen and therefore is worth preparing for. Sometimes, people will react with embarrassment, discomfort, or outright hostility once they learn that you have a hearing problem. People who are extremely shy might be embarrassed when talking to you, but they probably act this way because they are afraid they won't be able to converse well enough to make the grade, so to speak. The same type of person might stammer at a cocktail party when he's around people he doesn't know, and is afraid of being thought a poor conversationalist. If this is the case, a friendly attitude on your part will help put him at ease.

As far as blatant hostility, remember that when someone is hostile for no good reason, it's likely that person's problem, not yours. Sometimes, people who react with hostility when you tell them about your hearing loss suspect the same problem in themselves, but are afraid to own up to it, and subconsciously try to reject their own problem by being nasty to you. To be frank, someone who displays this type of animosity—or any sort of prejudice toward you—might not be worth communicating with, anyway.

My hearing aid doesn't help at all in noisy situations. What can I do? It may be best to turn the volume down or just to shut it off. As explained in Chapter 6, hearing aids don't function well in background noise. Many experienced users find that in extremely difficult situations it's easier to avoid the distraction of the aid and rely entirely on speechreading skills.

A friend of mine who's had a hearing problem for years tells me she always tries to deal with male clerks and tellers because they are easier to understand than women. Do men speak better for some reason? No, but you may *hear* them better. Because of the nature of sound, it is easier to

understand low-pitched voices than high-pitched voices. You may, therefore, have an easier time understanding a man. Probably the hardest person
for you to understand will be a child or young teenager; in addition to
having higher-pitched voices than adults, they often are not particularly
careful with their articulation.

[14]
Money Problems

There's a good possibility that you are concerned about the typical hearing aid prices that were mentioned earlier. Well, your reaction is perfectly natural. There's no question that hearing aids are expensive, and most people—when they first learn how much an aid will cost—react by asking, "Isn't there some program that will help pay for this?"

Unfortunately, these people are usually disappointed. Medicare, the federal program you've been paying into for quite some time, won't pay for anything to do with the eventual purchase of a hearing aid. Medicare will pay for a hearing test if it is used in the diagnosis of a medical problem, but not for any testing done that is connected with a hearing aid. So be sure that any bill you submit for the hearing test does not mention the words "hearing aid."

Medicaid, on the other hand, may help in certain cases. The program is administered by the individual states, and varies widely among individual jurisdictions. In some states, Medicaid may provide payment for the hearing evaluation and some assistance toward the purchase of an aid, along with a limited amount of follow-up care. Other states, though, won't provide a thing.

How do you find out what your state's Medicaid system will pay for? First, look in the listing of state offices in your phone book; you will almost certainly find a listing for "social services." Call this department and ask for information about Medicaid coverage. If you don't find that listing, or a similar one, try the state's general information number, usually found at the beginning of the listings. If that doesn't help, ask your audiologist.

Don't get your hopes up about Medicaid, by the way. As noted earlier, your state may not have any benefits related to buying a hearing aid. With the current cost-cutting fervor, existing government benefits may be modified or cut back altogether. (This is why a listing of state-by-state benefits was not included in this book. These programs are currently in a state of flux, and any information gathered at the time of this writing could be inaccurate shortly after the first printing.) Also, keep in mind that you must meet certain low-income standards to qualify for Medicaid benefits, and the required investigation of your personal finances can be a demeaning process.

If you haven't yet reached retirement age, check into your state's vocational rehabilitation program (see Chapter 13). These are designed for people who are still of working age but who have lost a job or have trouble keeping a job because of a handicap. Vocational rehabilitation programs may, in some cases, help pay for a hearing aid and provide counseling and job retraining. Like Medicaid, vocational rehabilitation programs are being modified, and also vary widely from state to state. To find out what's available in your locality, scan the state-office telephone listings for any department with the word "vocational" or "rehabilitation" in the title. If this doesn't work, call the social services office, or ask your audiologist for help.

Private insurers who pay for hearing aids are scarce indeed. Only a handful of very large corporations have health insurance plans that could cover the cost of getting a hearing aid and learning to use it. In most cases, your policy probably won't pay for costs related to a hearing loss, but it never hurts to check. Call your insurer or company personnel office to find out for sure.

In a few special cases, local fraternal groups, such as the Lions or Kiwanis, may pay for part or all of an individual's hearing aid cost. However, this is done on a case-by-case basis. If you think there is a compelling reason why one of these organizations would want to help, apply, by all means.

There aren't too many other possibilities for finding money to pay for your hearing aid. But even though there is not much in the way of financial assistance, you can help yourself by shopping wisely and not spending money you don't have to. If you do end up paying the bill, don't forget that the whole cost is tax deductible as a medical expense.

Because a hearing aid is a substantial investment, you will want to protect it. Some guidelines for extending the life of your aid are contained in Chapter 6. Another helpful hint is to have the aid reconditioned when, after a few years, it develops common wear-related problems. When an aid is reconditioned, the dispenser ships it to the factory, where technicians replace most of the internal workings. Cost of reconditioning depends on the age of the aid, but on a three-year-old aid, for example, reconditioning will generally run less than a hundred dollars. After reconditioning, you've essentially got a new instrument in your old case, and it may last for five more years.

As mentioned earlier, you can often save money on services related to a hearing aid (fitting the aid, or hearing-therapy sessions, for instance) by finding a college-sponsored clinic in your area. Rates will undoubtedly be considerably lower than those charged in nontraining facilities. You will, in most cases, be working with students; these students are under the direct supervision of a qualified audiologist. The only problem you're likely to encounter is that students need more time to conduct tests than experienced audiologists do. But if you've got the extra time to spend, the college clinic will be well worth it.

Although college audiology clinics may help with hearing tests and therapy, you won't be able to avoid that required trip to the physician, as discussed in Chapter 7, nor should you try. It is essential to be sure that there's no dangerous medical problem causing your hearing loss. (It's unlikely that there is one, but you're better off playing it safe.)

A visit to the doctor may be covered by your health insurance, but not by Medicare, if the examination is in preparation for a hearing aid. If the physician's appraisal is not covered by your insurer, you can save some money by scheduling the exam at a public clinic. In any event, expect a hefty fee for a visit to any specialist, especially if it's your first time at the office. The visit to the doctor is an unavoidable expense, as is much of the hearing aid process.

Perhaps, then, you feel that this chapter has added up to a big, fat zero because it doesn't offer any magic formula for getting financial aid. Unfortunately, it is true that almost any other health problem is dealt with by more social and/or public assistance programs. However, if you add up the costs and balance them against what you are really paying for, you may not feel so bad. When you shell out something like $500 for a hearing aid, you are actually purchasing another sense, an ability to communicate. You will use your hearing aid far more often than the family car, and will certainly get better mileage from it.

Some of the money you spend for an aid also goes toward research and development by the hearing aid manufacturer, in much the same way as part of the price of gasoline pays for the oil companies' exploration for new petroleum deposits. This added cost is considerable, but judging by the recent great advances in hearing aid technology, it is well worth it.

There's also a question of supply and demand. Companies just don't sell that many hearing aids, and because few units are sold, the individual price remains high. Basically, this situation exists because only a fraction of the people who need hearing aids actually buy them. If it's any consolation, by deciding to take the plunge and buy one of today's relatively expensive hearing aids, you've become part of the solution to the overall money problem.

The next chapter will conclude our exploration of coping with hearing loss. First, some typical questions on money matters:

I'm pretty handy at fixing my radio. If something goes wrong with my aid, can I try and save money by fixing it myself? A thousand times, no! Unless you are an electronic engineer with a laboratory full of equipment, you don't stand a chance of being able to fix the aid. You will only damage it further and make the repair bill even worse, and will probably also invalidate the manufacturer's warranty. Take it back to the dispenser and stick to fixing radios.

I've seen mail order ads for hearing aids. Should I consider buying one of these? Because hearing aids are supposed to be individually prescribed to deal with specific hearing disorders, there's little chance that any instrument purchased through the mail will come close to fitting your needs. The earmold that comes with it won't be an exact fit, as would a custom-made model. Also, you won't get necessary services and adjustments when you order an aid through the mail, so what seems like a good bargain probably isn't.

I'm not sure I can come up with the money for a hearing aid all in one chunk. Can I buy one on installment? Some hearing aid dispensers will allow you to pay over a period of time; the only way to find out is by asking. If you are expected to pay interest, ask for a clear and direct explanation of the interest rate, and be sure to find out the total amount you'll have to pay.

[15]
Coping

One thing that often puzzles doctors and audiologists is the common reaction of people who are told they have a hearing loss. "Oh God," they say, "do I have to wear a hearing aid?"

No, of course they don't *have* to—but isn't that entirely the wrong attitude, anyway? If you feel that way—if you dread the thought of having your suspicions confirmed by a hearing test, or of wearing the hearing aid you know you need, or having to live with a permanent hearing loss—stop and think for a moment. Wouldn't it be better if you looked at it this way?

JUST A FEW YEARS AGO, VERY LITTLE COULD BE DONE FOR PEOPLE WITH HEARING LOSSES. TODAY, THERE ARE CONCERNED PROFESSIONALS WHO CAN HELP ME REGAIN A SENSE.

We hope that this book has given you the motivation to do something constructive about your hearing loss. We hope, too, that you will conclude that while a hearing loss means that things will change, those things don't always have to change for the worse. Coping with a hearing loss means altering your environment when and where you can. You may have to rearrange the furniture in the living room in order to see your guests' faces more clearly. Does this mean that since your living room must be different, it must be worse? No, of course not. The same type of reasoning applies to most of the new lifestyle you must adopt to deal with your hearing loss.

It's not all as simple as rearranging the furniture, of course, and you will have to live within certain limitations. But by polishing your communication skills and emotionally accepting the problem, you can keep those limitations to a minimum. There's a tendency for people with a hearing loss to let it grow all out of proportion in the total scheme of things. Sometimes, the hearing loss becomes the dominant force in their lives—with every depressing minute spent thinking of how much better things would be "if I only didn't have something wrong with me."

Well, *there's nothing wrong with you*. There's something wrong with your ears, of course, but your ears are just a small part of all the things that are *you*. You'll have to come up with your own formula for evaluating self-worth; perhaps you value your honesty, or pride yourself on a lifetime of accomplishment and hard work. But whatever you use to gauge your self-worth, the state of your hearing should play no part of it.

In fact, there's something to be said for dealing with adversity; because of your lifetime of experience, you certainly know this. That makes you better able to cope with your hearing loss and emerge a stronger person.

Unfortunately, there are people who just don't feel up to the challenge of meeting the problem head-on. If you're tempted to take this attitude, remember that you are not the only one who will be affected. If you suffer, so do the people who love you. If you punish yourself, you punish them, too, for it will hurt them to see you depressed, isolated, and lonely.

Throughout this book, we've stressed the fact that a hearing loss is a common problem; millions of people are in the same boat as you. But don't interpret this as meaning that you should decide not to do anything about it. Bad backs are common too, but if you developed a painful back, chances are you would try to get it taken care of as quickly as possible.

Plenty of people, young and old, haven't let hearing problems slow them down: President Ronald Reagan, actress Nanette Fabray, and comedian Norm Crosby are a few examples. Actor Keenan Wynn has had a distinguished career, including appearances in TV's "Dallas," despite a hearing loss. Bodybuilder Lou Ferrigno, who came to fame as "The Incredible Hulk," has had a severe hearing loss from childhood, but he never let it stop him from becoming one of the strongest men in the world and a performer on network television—a performer who has handled a variety of roles and who has acted as a spokesman for a hearing-help organization.

These people found that there was help available, and they took advantage of it. You can, too.

Glossary

Air Conduction: Transmission of sound to the inner ear by way of the ear canal and the middle ear.

Anvil: The middle bone of the three bones (ossicles) in the middle ear that transmit sound vibration. (Latin *incus*.)

Assertiveness: Behavior that allows people to request their own rights without interfering with the rights of others.

Audiologist: (aud ee OL oh jist): A person who holds a degree and/or certification in the areas of identification and measurement of hearing impairments, and rehabilitation of persons with hearing impairments.

Auditory nerve (AUD i tor ee): The cranial nerve carrying information from the inner ear to the brain.

Aural rehabilitation (AUR al): Educational/therapeutic procedures used with hearing-impaired persons to improve the effectiveness of their overall communication ability.

Binaural aids (bine AUR al): Two separate amplification systems worn simultaneously on two separate ears of the individual.

Bone conduction: Transmission of sound to the inner ear by applying vibration to the bones of the skull.

Cerumen (sair ROO men): Wax that is produced in the ear canal.

Closed-captioned television: Printed text shown on the television screen for certain shows when an adaptor is attached to the television.

Closure (CLOZE yure): The ability to recognize a whole when one or more of the parts are missing.

Cochlea (COKE lee uh): The hearing part of the inner ear, which resembles a snail shell.

Communication disorders: Any interference with an individual's ability to comprehend or express ideas, experiences, knowledge, or feelings.

Conductive hearing loss: A deficit in hearing caused by an abnormality in the outer or middle ear.

Decibel: A measure of the intensity (loudness) of a sound.

Discrimination *(acoustics):* The degree to which one is able to hear and recognize differences among the speech sounds, i.e., the ability to understand speech once it is loud enough to hear.

Dispensing audiologist: An audiologist who sells and fits hearing aids, as well as evaluates hearing and provides aural rehabilitation.

Eardrum: A thin, concave, parchmentlike membrane that stretches across the ear canal and separates the outer ear from the middle ear.

Earmold: A plasticlike fitting in the outer ear, designed to transmit the amplified sound from a hearing aid into the ear.

ENT specialist: A person who holds a degree in medicine and who specializes in the treatment of problems associated with the ear, nose, and throat. Also called otolaryngologist or head and neck surgeon.

Eustachean tube (yus TASHE an): An air duct from the area back of the nose to the middle ear.

Feedback *(acoustics):* Sound that escapes from the receiver of a hearing aid or other amplification system and reaches the microphone, producing a squealing sound.

Footplate: The base of the stirrup, which rests on the oval window.

Frequency *(acoustics)*: A measure of the pitch of a sound.

Hair cells: The sensory receptors in the inner ear that translate the sound vibration into messages that go into the brain.

Hammer: The first and largest of the three bones (ossicles) in the middle ear that transmit sound vibrations. (Latin *malleus.*)

Hearing aid dealer: A person who sells and fits hearing aids. Some dealers prefer to be called dispensers.

Hearing aid dispenser: A person who sells and fits hearing aids.

Hearing aid evaluation: A process of determining if one or more hearing aids is appropriate, and what type of amplification system would help to utilize the patient's residual hearing.

Hearing ear dog: A dog that is trained to alert its hearing-impaired master to auditory signals such as doorbells, smoke alarms, wake-up alarms, baby cries, etc.

Hearing evaluation: A measure of the capability of a person's auditory system to perceive and interpret sound. A determination of the extent and type of hearing loss.

Hearing screening: A gross measure to separate out those persons who require special help for a hearing problem.

Hearing therapist: An audiologist or speech-language pathologist who provides aural rehabilitation.

Homophonous (ho MOF en us): When sounds look identical on the lips when produced by a speaker.

Impedance measurements: A physical measurement of a sound reflected off the eardrum and analyzed to reveal characteristics of the middle ear.

Inner ear: The interior section of the ear where sound vibrations and body positions (balance) are transformed into nerve impulses.

Lipreading: *See* speechreading.

Meniere's disease (min YARES): An overaccumulation of fluid in the inner ear causing a fluctuating hearing loss, dizziness, roaring sounds in the ear, and a feeling of fullness in the head and ears.

Middle ear: The section of the ear extending from the eardrum to the oval window.

Nerve deafness: A misleading term often used to describe a sensorineural hearing loss.

Ossicles (OSS i culls): The tiny bones in the middle ear that transmit the sound vibrations. They are known as the hammer, anvil, and stirrup, and are listed individually in this glossary.

Otitis media (oh TITE is MEE dee uh): Inflammation of the middle ear, usually caused by infection.

Otologist (oh TOL oh jist): A person who holds a medical degree and specializes in problems of the ears.

Otoscope (OH toe scope): An instrument for visual examination of the ear canal and eardrum.

Ototoxic (oh toe TOX ic): Poisonous to the ear—usually referring to drugs.

Outer ear: The funnellike structure for receiving sound; it includes the pinna, the ear canal, and the eardrum.

Oval window: A membrane, the resting place of the stirrup, which pulsates with vibrations of the middle ear and transmits them into the fluid of the inner ear.

Pinna (PIN uh): The part of the ear that is visible on the outside of the head.

Presbycusis (pres bi CUSE is): Hearing loss due to the aging process.

Pure tone (acoustics): A sound at only one frequency (pitch) with no harmonics.

Recruitment (re CROOT ment): A phenomenon sometimes accompanying a sensorineural hearing loss in which a slight increase in the intensity of a sound results in a disproportionate increase in the sensation of loudness, causing oversensitivity to loud sounds.

Resonance (REZ oh nance): The vibration of an object or a body of air where certain pitches are made louder; this is the effect noted in blowing over the top of a bottle.

Semicircular canals: Three looped bony tubes in the ear that help to maintain a sense of balance.

Sensitivity (acoustics): Ability to react to varying degrees of a stimulus such as sound.

Sensorineural hearing loss (sen sor ee NOOR al): A deficit in hearing caused by an abnormality in the inner ear or the auditory nerve.

Speech pathology: Also known as speech-language pathology. The study of speech, language, and voice disorders for the purposes of diagnosis and treatment.

Speechreading: Utilization of nonauditory cues to comprehend what is being spoken. Also called lipreading.

Speech reception threshold: The softest intensity level at which an individual can recognize speech.

Speech therapist: A person who has a degree and/or certification in the areas of diagnosing speech, language, and voice disorders, and of implementing therapeutic measures. Also called a speech-language pathologist.

Stirrup: The third and smallest bone (ossicle) in the middle ear that transmits sound vibrations. (Latin *stapes*.)

TDD: *See* telecommunications device for the deaf.

Telecommunications device for the deaf (abbreviated TDD): A telephone system for the severely hearing impaired where a typewritten message is transmitted over the telephone lines and is received as a visual message. One type of TDD is a teletypewriter (TTY).

Tinnitus (TIN ih tus or ti NIGH tus): A ringing or roaring sensation in the head or ears, which may be a result of auditory impairment.

Tinnitus masker: A hearing aid–like device that produces a noise that covers up the internal ringing, buzzing, or roaring sounds experienced by many hearing-impaired people.

T-switch: An adjustment device on a hearing aid with an inductance wire so that the aid can pick up electromagnetic waves from a telephone receiver or a group amplification system.

Tympanum: The tympanic membrane (eardrum) or cavity (middle ear).

Vocational rehabilitation: Evaluation and retraining for employment when a disability prevents a person from doing a previous job.

Volume wheel: An adjustable device to make a sound louder or softer; often found on hearing aids or telephone receivers.

Word recognition testing: Measurement of an individual's ability to understand words once the words are loud enough.

Index